Acclaim for

POWER FOODS FOR THE BRAIN

"This is a book everyone should read from a doctor whose advice I trust. POWER FOODS FOR THE BRAIN will help you maximize your brain power and prevent problems down the road concerning memory loss. Buy it now before you forget to."

—Ellen DeGeneres

"A timely and critically important book on a topic that will be of concern to many people."

—T. Colin Campbell, PhD, professor emeritus, Cornell University, co-author of *The China Study*

"This is a game changer for anyone concerned with memory or cognition. The great news is that Dr. Barnard has, once again, given us the keys to prevention and profound healing, and those keys are easily accessible."

—Kathy Freston

"POWER FOODS FOR THE BRAIN shows the amazing ability that foods have to keep body and mind going strong...If you want to stay sharp and be your healthiest self, the information this book provides will get you there."

—Alicia Silverstone

"Simple changes to your diet and exercise can help you be at your best when you're young and help prevent memory problems when you're older. POWER FOODS FOR THE BRAIN shows you how, step-by-step...An immensely practical and important book."

—Dean Ornish, MD, founder and president, Preventive Medicine Research Institute, clinical professor of medicine, University of California, San Francisco

"Dr. Neal Barnard is one of the most responsible and authoritative voices in American medicine today."

—Andrew Weil, MD

"Simple, effective strategies for preventing dementias—not with drugs, but with great-tasting food and healthy lifestyle choices. Finally, a low-cost (and delicious) doctor's prescription you will enjoy filling—and one you'll be able to remember to refill, year after year! Given the tsunami of dementias bearing down upon our society, POWER FOODS FOR THE BRAIN is, potentially, one of the most important books of the decade."

—Michael Kapler, MD, director, Institute of Nutrition Education and Research, Manhattan Beach, CA

"Enhance your intellect with food. Dr. Barnard's simple dietary prescription also prevents strokes, Alzheimer's disease, and other causes of loss of mental function. The recipes are easy and delicious."

—John McDougall, MD, author and founder, McDougall Program

POWER FOODS
FOR THE BRAIN

ALSO BY NEAL D. BARNARD, MD

The Power of Your Plate

A Physician's Slimming Guide

Food for Life

Eat Right, Live Longer

Foods That Fight Pain

Turn Off the Fat Genes

Breaking the Food Seduction

Nutrition Guide for Clinicians

The Cancer Survivor's Guide

Dr. Neal Barnard's Program for Reversing Diabetes

21-Day Weight Loss Kickstart

POWER FOODS

FOR THE BRAIN

AN EFFECTIVE 3-STEP PLAN TO PROTECT
YOUR MIND AND STRENGTHEN YOUR MEMORY

Neal D. Barnard, MD

With Recipes by Christine Waltermyer
and Jason Wyrick

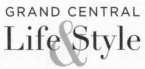

GRAND CENTRAL
Life & Style
NEW YORK · BOSTON

Grand Central Life & Style
Hachette Book Group
237 Park Avenue
New York, NY 10017
www.HachetteBookGroup.com

Printed in the United States of America

LSC-C

Originally published in hardcover by Grand Central Life & Style.

First trade edition: February 2014
10 9 8 7 6 5 4

Grand Central Life & Style is an imprint of Grand Central Publishing.
The Grand Central Life & Style name and logo are trademarks of Hachette Book Group, Inc.

The Hachette Speakers Bureau provides a wide range of authors for speaking events. To find out more, go to www.hachettespeakersbureau.com or call (866) 376-6591.

The publisher is not responsible for websites (or their content) that are not owned by the publisher.

The Library of Congress has cataloged the hardcover edition as follows:

Barnard, Neal D.
    Power foods for the brain : an effective 3-step plan to protect your mind and strengthen your memory / by Neal D. Barnard ; with recipes by Christine Waltermyer and Jason Wyrick. — 1st ed.
       p. cm.
    ISBN 978-1-4555-1219-5
    1. Functional foods. 2. Memory disorders — Prevention. 3. Nootropic agents.
4. Cooking. I. Waltermyer, Christine. II. Wyrick, Jason. III. Title.
    QP144.F85B37 2013
    616.8'3—dc23   2012013272

ISBN 978-1-4555-1220-1 (pbk.)

To Drs. David and Alexandra Jenkins,
who are lighting the way for others to follow.

Contents

Step III   DEFEAT MEMORY THREATS

PUTTING THE PLAN INTO ACTION

A Note to the Reader

I hope this book provides you with new insights into important health issues and gives you tools to tackle them. Before we begin, let me mention two important points:

See your health-care provider. Memory problems are serious business. It is important to have an appropriate evaluation and care. I would also encourage you to speak with your provider before making any diet change. This is not because changing your diet is necessarily dangerous. Quite the opposite. Adjusting the menu is a good idea. But people who are taking medications—for diabetes or high blood pressure, for example—very often need to adjust their medications when they improve their diets. Sometimes they are able to discontinue their drugs altogether. Do not do this on your own. Work with your health-care provider to reduce or discontinue medicines if and when the time is right.

Also, talk with your doctor before you jump into a new exercise routine. If you have been sedentary, have any serious health problems, have a great deal of weight to lose, or are over forty, have your provider check whether you are ready for exercise, and how rapidly to begin.

Get complete nutrition. The way of eating presented in this book is likely to improve your nutrition overall, in addition to the specific health benefits it may bring. Even so, you will want to ensure that you get complete nutrition. Please read the details in chapter 10. In particular, be sure to take a daily multiple vitamin or other reliable source of vitamin B_{12}, such as fortified cereals or fortified soy milk. Vitamin B_{12} is essential for healthy nerves and healthy blood.

Acknowledgments

I owe an enormous debt of gratitude to many people who helped bring this project to fruition. First, thanks to our research team and colleagues who, over the years, have shaped fundamental concepts of health and nutrition: Mark Sklar, MD; Andrew Nicholson, MD; Gabrielle Turner-McGrievy, PhD; Joshua Cohen, MD; Kavita Rajasekhar, MD; Ulka Agarwal, MD; Suruchi Mishra, PhD; Paul Poppen, PhD; Susan Levin, MS, RD; Joseph Gonzales, RD; Jia Xu, PhD; Heather Katcher, PhD; Lisa Gloede, RD; Ernest Noble, MD; Jill Eckart, CHHC; and Amber Green, RD.

Thanks also to the many investigators at other research centers whose work has brought to light the power of foods to affect health in general and the brain in particular. I am particularly grateful to Martha Clare Morris, ScD, of Rush University Medical Center, whose painstaking work has opened up new possibilities for protecting the brain. David J. A. Jenkins, MD, PhD, of the University of Toronto, continues to lead groundbreaking nutrition research with direct benefits for countless people.

Christine Waltermyer and Jason Wyrick used their considerable culinary skills to turn the scientific concepts in this book into wonderful recipes.

John McDougall, MD, and Mary McDougall have been constant

inspirations and fountains of information, and answered many questions along the way.

Special thanks to the physicians, scientists, and others who critically reviewed the manuscript: Lawrence A. Hansen, MD; Erika D. Driver-Dunckley, MD; Travis Dunckley, PhD; Leonid Shkolnik, MD; Clifford Schostal, MD; Nikhil Kulkarni, MD; Hope Ferdowsian, MD; Caroline Trapp, MSN, APRN, BC-ADM, CDE; Edie Broida, MS; Brenda Davis, RD; Doug Hall; Lynn Maurer; Shaina Chimes; and Jillian Gibson.

Thank you to Ellsworth Wareham, MD, and Duane Graveline, MD, for allowing me to share their experiences and profit from their wisdom. Thank you to Cael Croft for his excellent illustrations and to Chris Evans, PhD, of the University of Glamorgan, Wales, for helping me color the manuscript with historical facts.

Huge thanks to my editor, Diana Baroni, and my literary agent, Debra Goldstein, for their enthusiastic support and expertise in transforming concepts and ideas into a tangible tool that can be put to work for better health.

And finally, thank you to everyone at the Physicians Committee for Responsible Medicine for your boundless innovation and energy in spreading the word about good health.

Introduction

They were not very tidy and not very clean....They
smoked as they played and they ate and talked and
pretended to hit each other. They turned their backs
on the audience and shouted at them and laughed
at private jokes.[1]

That was how Brian Epstein described the Beatles when he
first saw them at a Liverpool club in 1961. In leather jackets
and jeans, this ragtag foursome did not attract the interest of a
single record company in Britain, or anyone else outside a short
radius.

Yes, they were scruffy. But they had energy and magnetism,
and plenty of drive and ambition. They couldn't read music, but
they had an irresistible sound. Although Epstein had never managed a band before, he took them under his wing, determined
to help them succeed. He dragged them to a London tailor and
plunked down £40. Out with the leather jackets and jeans and
in with proper suits. And no more "greaser" haircuts; it was time
for a new hairstyle. No eating, smoking, or swearing onstage,
and please learn to bow to the audience at the end of a set.
He scheduled performances, arranged publicity, and made sure
everyone got paid.

Within nine months, the Beatles had their first hit on the British pop charts, and within two years, they had conquered the world.

The reason I am telling you this is because inside your brain you have unruly needs, wants, drives, and ambitions, too. Your "early Beatles" reside deep in the center of your brain, in your hypothalamus. This nut-size organ is the locus of hunger, thirst, sex, and anger. And if there is one thing it needs, it is a manager.

By the time you were born, your hypothalamus was already signaling its demands. But all you could do about it was to wail and thrash your arms and legs.

Your "Brian Epstein" is in the outer layers of your brain, in your cerebral cortex. It takes your ragtag, scruffy self and all its wants, drives, and ambitions, and gets things organized. It helps the desperate hypothalamus to wait patiently when food is on the way. It solves your problems and guides you to get what you want more effectively than by simply stamping your feet. As the years go by, your manager matures, developing ever more sophisticated ways of getting what you need and like.

By August 27, 1967, eighteen Beatles songs had topped the charts, and they were at the peak of their popularity. But that was the day that everything changed. Brian Epstein was found dead in his apartment. He was just thirty-two. And for the Beatles, it was the beginning of the end. The group began to sputter. They had arguments, with no arbiter. Disagreements became chronic and bitter. Rudderless, they lost their musical cohesiveness, drifted apart, and eventually the most successful musical group of all time collapsed, each member going his own way.

Inside your brain, your own fateful August 27 is looming large. Just when your knowledge and experience are at their maximum and your family life and perhaps your financial security are finally established, that's exactly the moment that you are at risk of losing your manager. If that happens, you will find that you can't remember things or will have trouble reasoning things out. Sometimes things go downhill to the point where you are no longer able to control your disorganized, unruly, unmanaged inner self. The day the manager in your brain becomes nonfunctional is the day that life as you have known it comes to an end.

This is a book about keeping your manager alive and well. It is about memory and mental clarity, and keeping them intact lifelong.

What's Happening in My Brain?

It starts as an occasional lapse. You've forgotten a name or word—something you know perfectly well but just cannot put your finger on. Later on, it happens again, and you start to wonder what's wrong. Maybe you're overtired or overstressed, and a good night's sleep will set everything to rights.

But maybe it is more than that. Memory problems affect a great many people. They are worrying, to say the least. Not being able to come up with a friend's name, losing your keys one too many times, losing track of facts and events, and, perhaps worst of all, having others *notice* that you seem to be having trouble—none of this is good.

It may not be just memory. Sometimes you might feel that your thinking is just not as clear as it used to be. You'll be adding up your checkbook or reading a newspaper article and you'll feel as if your brain is stuck in low gear.

And sometimes cognitive problems are very serious. One in five Americans between the ages of seventy-five and eighty-four develops Alzheimer's disease. Beyond age eighty-five, it hits almost half of us. Also frighteningly common are strokes, which can devastate our ability to speak, move, and think.

Of all the worries we may have about our future, the possibility of losing our mental abilities tops the list. We work hard, start our families, set aside some money, and finally have some time to relax and enjoy life. But if memory loss enters the scene, it steals everything we cherish.

Losing our memory and brainpower means stripping away our most critical capabilities. Little by little, we start to slip away from our families. Things we did together are erased. If the process drags on over years, as it often does, it can end up encumbering our families and eventually exhausting them physically, emotionally, and financially.

A poor memory is not just "a part of life" that you have to put up with. And it is certainly not an automatic part of growing older. Your calendar does not come equipped with an eraser.

Imagine having a sharp memory—and good concentration and alertness—day after day for as long as you live. Instead of apologizing for names that elude you, the words come easily, just as they always did. Instead of lapsing into memory problems in older age, your mind remains clear and strong.

For many years, my research team has been investigating the role of foods in health. We have helped people trim away weight and cut their cholesterol levels. We developed a dietary method for managing diabetes that is more powerful than previous diets, sometimes making the disease essentially disappear. We have also developed programs for the workplace and for doctors' offices, designed to help people make diet changes to improve their health.

Just as we were doing our studies, other research teams were looking at the brain and how specific nutritional factors could affect the risk of Alzheimer's disease, stroke, and other serious brain problems, as well as the surprising effects of foods on more day-to-day cognitive issues.

In Chicago, researchers from Rush University Medical Center have been tracking thousands of people, teasing apart what separates those who stay healthy and sharp throughout life from those who don't, finding that particular aspects of diet and lifestyle are key. Other researchers in the United States, Europe, and Asia have conducted detailed studies into specific nutrients that either protect or attack the brain. Meanwhile, new brain scanning techniques have allowed researchers to look into the brains of living human beings to understand brain function in ways that were impossible even a few years ago. Special tests have begun to show who is at risk for cognitive problems as the years go by.

Along the way, it has become clear that the diet changes my research team found to promote physical health and those that other researchers have found to be critical for brain health are remarkably similar. Specific foods and eating patterns have a powerful protective effect.

And there is more to it. It is possible to exercise the brain in simple ways that, over time, strengthen the connections between brain cells. And simple physical exercises actually allow you to counteract the brain shrinking that occurs in most people as they age.

It is urgent that people know about these findings, and that is why I've written this book and developed this program. The fact is, we know more than ever about how our memory works and about the causes of memory problems, whether they are minor lapses, "senior moments," or potentially devastating problems like Alzheimer's disease and stroke. And yet most people have no idea of any of this. While they may have a pretty clear idea about how to prevent lung cancer and how to reduce their risk of heart attack, most have absolutely no clue that it is possible to protect the brain.

There are simple, powerful steps that you can take, starting right now. This book will show you how to put this information to work and help preserve your memory and strengthen your brain.

Three Steps to Protect Your Brain

Taking advantage of what research has shown is not difficult. Here are three steps you can take that will shield your brain:

Step One: The first step is using power foods to give your brain the nutrition it needs. We will select foods with three things in mind:

First, we'll shield you from toxins that are in everyday foods and water. They are surprisingly common, and it is critical to know where they are and how to avoid them.

Second, certain natural fats are essential for brain function, while others are harmful. We'll see which are which and where they are on your plate. The correct balance makes a big difference in helping each brain cell work optimally.

Third, certain vitamins knock out free radicals and other compounds that could damage brain cells. We'll see which foods and supplements provide the nutrients you need.

Building a healthful menu is the most important thing you can do. After all, every minute of the day, your brain cells are bathing in the nutrients—or toxins—you've taken in through foods.

Step Two: Did you know you can exercise your brain? Simple mental exercises strengthen connections within your brain. They are surprisingly easy, fun, and powerful. I'll help you develop a regimen for peak performance.

Physical exercises are powerful, too. Just as exercise strengthens your heart, it does the same for your brain. The effect of physical exercise is so dramatic that MRI scans can demonstrate a visible difference in brain structure in a relatively short period of time. You'll learn which exercises are most helpful to the brain and why.

Step Three: Now it's time to defeat the common physical threats to your memory and preserve and enhance your brain. There are two specific issues you'll want to address: sleep disruptions and certain medications and medical conditions.

Sleep is essential for integrating memories, and many cognitive problems can be traced to common sleep disruptions. We will see how to correct any problems so you can take advantage of the natural integrative power of sleep.

Common medications and medical conditions can derail your thought processes, sometimes to the point of being mistaken for Alzheimer's disease—until the cause is identified. I'll show you the surprising list of common culprits and what to do about them.

Whether you aim to simply boost your brainpower, eliminate daily lapses, or cut your risk of Alzheimer's disease and stroke, you will want to put each of these simple steps to work so you can be at your absolute best for the long haul. Implementing your brain-enhancing strategy will be easy with the advice I offer and the menu plans and delicious recipes I'll share.

Time for a Change

Millions of families are worried about what the future holds for them. During my training in neurology and psychiatry at the George Washington University School of Medicine in Washington, D.C., I had my first encounters with patients who felt that their minds and nervous systems were no longer their own. Some were succumbing to severe memory loss caused by

Alzheimer's. Others had had strokes. And still others showed the progressive nerve symptoms caused by multiple sclerosis or other conditions. There was very little we could do to help them and nothing we knew of that could prevent these problems from arising.

Even today, most people—including many doctors—have yet to learn about the techniques you will read about here. And even though the medications that aim to slow the onslaught of memory problems are all but useless, few doctors and patients have learned about the new research on the power of nutrition. Most have no idea that their mealtime choices could make a difference.

This book changes that. The fact is, there is much we can do to prevent memory loss, not to mention maximize the everyday function of people who simply want to feel their best.

Simple choices can enhance and protect your brain, give you energy, improve your sleep, and boost your overall health. I will show you how.

Science Thrives on Controversy

Not long ago someone gave me a book on survival in wilderness settings. It helpfully pointed out that if you happened to wash up on some faraway island in the middle of nowhere, a wild Malay apple would be perfectly safe to eat, while the fruit of the *pangi* tree could kill you. If you found an ordinary strawberry, it would be delicious, but a look-alike *duchesnea* is poisonous. And it is important to be able to tell an edible Dryad's saddle mushroom from a deadly panther cap. After a few pages I realized I had no idea how to handle any such situation and was grateful to have a grocery store across the street.

Nutrition can be confusing, and, as a result, different people interpret things in different ways. When it comes to research on food and the brain, scientists all have their own opinions. Some want to wait before suggesting any diet changes. They feel we need more research before we can make definitive statements.

Others, including me, feel that we do not have the luxury of waiting. If you are planning your dinner this evening, you are stacking the odds one way or the other. You need to go by the best information available. As you'll see, that information is powerful and is easy to put into action. At least it's easier than trying to identify the fruit of the *pangi* tree.

All the Side Effects Are Good Ones

As you put the findings of this book to work to protect your brain, you may notice not only that you feel mentally sharp. You may also find that your bathroom scale is becoming friendlier day by day. Your cholesterol and blood pressure may improve, and if you have diabetes, it may get better, too. If you have arthritis or other chronic aches and pains, you may notice that they are fading. That's the power of healthful eating.

My hope is that, instead of searching for words or worrying about your memory, you'll be searching for a tougher crossword puzzle, calling up old schoolmates whose names you remember well, and planning your next walking trip through the Rockies.

I hope you enjoy the very best of health and all the foods that will bring it to you.

POWER
FOODS
FOR THE BRAIN

CHAPTER 1

Sharpen Your Memory, Enhance Your Brain

In my previous books on health and nutrition, I have translated the research findings of my team and others into steps to help people conquer diabetes, cholesterol problems, chronic pain, and other health concerns. However, this book did not start with our research studies. It started with my own family.

My mother's father was a physician in a small Iowa town back when house calls and home births were everyday parts of a doctor's work. His diet, like that of the rest of the family, was typical Iowa fare, which is to say it was long on meat and potatoes and short on green vegetables and fruits. Long before the advent of health insurance, patients did not always have money to pay for his services. So people often paid with a chicken or a cut of beef.

At around age sixty, he suffered his first heart attack. And not long after that, his behavior started to change. He became confused. Sometimes he set out for walks without seeming to know where he was going. Cars had to stop as he wandered across busy streets. Once in a while, a motorist knew him and brought him back home. With time, things got worse. He became aggressive and was put into a hospital, where another heart attack eventually killed him.

We never knew if his problems were due to Alzheimer's disease, a series of strokes, or something else. His wife, my grandmother, lived longer, but her memory went, too. "By the time I get to the end of an article in the newspaper, I've forgotten the beginning," she told me. Memory gaps here and there began to coalesce into ever-bigger caverns where she was unable to find her way. It was tragically downhill from there, as she fell into severe dementia.

Both of my father's parents suffered the same fate—a gradual decline into more and more severe cognitive problems to the point where they were essentially unresponsive to the world around them. They existed this way for years before finally dying.

Fast-forward. Not long after I got out of medical school, I became concerned about my mother. Her memory was fine at the time. It was her cholesterol that was a problem. She and my father lived in Fargo, North Dakota, where they and their five children took full advantage of a typical Midwestern diet, and the results showed up on her cholesterol test.

A diet change would have helped, but it was a tough sell for my dear, stubborn mom. It was not until her personal physician threatened to put her on cholesterol-lowering medication for the rest of her life that she decided to try some changes in the kitchen. And, to her credit, she eventually did throw out the cholesterol-laden meat, dairy products, eggs, and greasy foods, adopting a vegan diet for seven weeks before going back to see her doctor. And her doctor could not believe the change. Her cholesterol had dropped nearly 80 points, which he thought *had* to be the result of some kind of mistake in the laboratory! But the effect was real, and my mother no longer needed medicines at all.

She continued on a healthy diet and lured my father into healthier eating habits, too. At family get-togethers, my mother and I prepared healthful foods and did our best to rebuff the contributions of family members who remained loyal to our not-so-healthful North Dakota traditions.

Sometime later, my parents moved into a retirement home. And there healthy diets were not the order of the day. The management felt that people in their "golden years" were not interested in healthful eating, and meaty, cheesy fare was on the menu at every meal. My parents soon drifted back into unhealthful diets, and she and my father dug into whatever foods were in front of them.

My mother's cholesterol skyrocketed again. As time went by she developed a severe blockage in one of the carotid arteries that lead to the brain. And she began to complain that her memory was going.

My father started to have memory problems, too. As they became more severe, he had a battery of medical tests, none of which showed any treatable cause. His dementia worsened, and eventually he became expressionless, nearly mute, and immobile.

Were my family's problems all genetic? Or did the blame go to their Midwestern diet, or perhaps a lack of exercise? Were they missing out on the vital nutrients that protect the brain?

At that time, none of us had a clue about how to protect the brain. Even today, most people—including many doctors—have never learned about the nutritional steps or exercises that shore up brain function and cut the risk of memory loss. That is why I wrote this book.

Let me give you a quick overview of where we're headed.

Connections

Did you ever wonder how you remember a name, a face, a fact, or a song? Or how your brain holds on to all the coordinated movements it takes to ride a bicycle or drive a car so that it's all second nature? How do we remember the layout of our home or our neighborhood?

When your brain lays down a new memory trace, it does not create a new brain cell—a neuron—to stuff a fact into. Rather, it makes new connections—called *synapses*—between brain cells. Or it strengthens existing connections. So a rickety one-lane bridge that could accommodate a pedestrian or two becomes a two-lane bridge, a four-lane bridge, or an eight-lane thoroughfare.

Your brain is taking in your experiences, making sense of them, and then deciding what it needs to hold on to and what it can let go of. Important events and emotional moments stay, while today's weather forecast, a restaurant phone number, and movie showtimes get pitched into the recycling bin.

Sleep plays a vital role in the process. That is when your brain integrates memories—carefully filing them away so you can retrieve them later.

Unfortunately, our brain circuits are fragile. They are easily knocked off-kilter by a lack of certain nutrients, poor sleep, or a medication side effect. And sometimes synapses break. You might have trouble finding a name or a word that you know is in your memory banks somewhere, if only you could figure out where. And for some people, memory problems become serious.

Memory Lapses

What if your memory is sputtering and misfiring? What if you're having lapses more frequently than normal?

If that is happening to you, it is important to know that there is a surprising range of things that can derail your memory and cloud your thinking—problems that are often easy to identify and treat. Sometimes it is as simple as correcting your sleep habits. Many people are chronically sleep-deprived, often without realizing it, with noticeable effects on their memory function.

Other times it's a question of looking at medications you may be taking. As we will see in chapter 8, common medications can throw a wrench into your gray matter. Sometimes a medication causes no problem when used by itself but causes all manner of problems when prescribed in combination with other drugs.

There are many medical problems that affect the brain, too, from vitamin deficiencies to thyroid problems. So you'll want to have a medical evaluation, and I'll show you what you need to look out for so you can correct the problem.

Mild Cognitive Impairment

If memory problems continue and no cause can be spotted, your doctor would label the problem *mild cognitive impairment*. This term refers to a situation in which you are doing fine in other respects—you're able to socialize, take care of yourself, and enjoy life—but your memory and thinking are not as sharp as they were. You might be a bit slower when it comes to paying bills or balancing your checkbook, and you might forget to pick up your dry cleaning. You may have trouble with names and words. You may also have trouble solving problems, planning ahead, or focusing your attention.

How can you tell whether mild cognitive impairment will turn into something more serious? The answer is, you can't at first. Only as time goes on does the picture become clearer.

Your doctor will want to track how you are doing over time. He or she is likely to give you some simple tests, such as asking you to memorize a name and address—John Smith, 103 Orchard Street, Springfield—and to recall it a few minutes later. Or he or she might show you three common objects—a pen, a stapler, and a book, for example—and place them around the room, asking you to remember each object and its location later on. What your doctor is looking at is your ability to learn and hold on to new information, because that is an indicator of how likely it is that more serious problems lie ahead.[1]

These quick tests sometimes are followed by more formal testing, which can be repeated as often as needed. Some researchers add special examinations to try to predict who might be headed for Alzheimer's disease. Drawing a sample of spinal fluid, they would look for two proteins, called *beta-amyloid 42* and *tau*.[1] A low level of beta-amyloid 42 suggests that beta-amyloid, which is linked to Alzheimer's disease, has been deposited in the brain. A high level of tau protein suggests that neurons have been damaged.

Using an MRI or other scanning methods, they can look for brain shrinkage (particularly in a part of the brain called the hippocampus), reduced brain activity, or signs that amyloid has been deposited in the brain.

If you have mild cognitive impairment, you'll want to use each of the steps in the following chapters to regain function if you can and to prevent further loss.

Frances and Mary Lou

Frances and her younger sister Mary Lou were born in Milwaukee, Wisconsin, and have lived there all their lives. They inherited a large grocery store from their parents and worked there throughout their careers, making a comfortable living.

Both reported that around the time they turned sixty, they felt less sharp than before. For Mary Lou, that meant memory problems, which worsened over time. She found that she would often draw a blank for names and sometimes could not remember the words for common objects. She also found that she was no longer the math wizard she had been as a youngster, and she was not as able to keep her attention focused. In part as a result of these problems, she retired from her job. As the years went by, she found these problems annoying, and her doctor labeled them mild cognitive impairment. However, the condition never deteriorated into Alzheimer's disease, and she still lives in the same house she has been in for the past four decades.

Frances's situation was different. She, too, noticed that it often took a bit longer to remember names, but she observed no other problems at all, and even her difficulty with names did not get any worse. She is now in her mid-eighties and still works in the same job in the family store.

Later on, we will look at what may have made the difference in these two women's experiences.

Alzheimer's Disease

Not everyone with mild cognitive impairment progresses to Alzheimer's disease, but many do. As we've seen, Alzheimer's is extremely common among older folks. But the fact is that we are now at a turning point in Alzheimer's disease research, with the emergence of what appear to be powerful tools for reducing the likelihood that you will develop it. Unfortunately, treatments for people who already have Alzheimer's are not at all what they should be, but research studies suggest an effective preventive strategy, which I'll lay out for you in the next several chapters.

When Alzheimer's disease takes hold, it attacks your brain's centers for learning, memory, reasoning, and language.[2] Here are the common symptoms:

- **Difficulty learning and remembering new things.** You might misplace personal belongings more frequently than normal. You might ask the same questions repeatedly, or get lost on what had been a familiar route.
- **Poor reasoning, judgment, or problem solving.** It becomes harder to make decisions, plan activities, handle routine finances, or take the usual steps to protect yourself (e.g., looking out for traffic before crossing a street).
- **Poor visuospatial abilities.** You might have trouble recognizing faces or using simple objects, or find it harder than it should be to do routine things like putting on your shoes or doing up buttons.
- **Losing language skills.** Words may elude you, and reading and writing can be more difficult.
- **Personality changes.** You could become irritable, agitated, or eventually just apathetic.

Alzheimer's is different from mild cognitive impairment in that cognitive problems are no longer just a nuisance; they are now interfering with your day-to-day activities. To reach the diagnosis, a doctor would look for at least two of the above symptoms. Typically these changes come on insidiously, unlike the more sudden cognitive problems caused by a stroke, trauma, or infection.

To separate Alzheimer's disease from other brain conditions, your doctor will do a physical exam and laboratory tests, and will also test your ability to learn and remember and can check your language skills. Sometimes doctors check cerebrospinal fluid, drawn via spinal tap, for *beta-amyloid 42* and *tau*. Special brain scans can spot amyloid deposits in the brain or shrinkage or reduced function in certain parts of the brain.

But even with sophisticated testing, your doctor cannot be entirely sure of the diagnosis. If it looks like Alzheimer's, the diagnosis will be called "possible" or "probable." A definitive diagnosis relies on an examination of the brain itself.

A Look Inside the Brain

If you were to look within the brain of a person with Alzheimer's disease, you would not find normal, healthy brain tissue. Here and there between the brain cells are tiny deposits of beta-amyloid protein. Doctors refer to these deposits as *plaques*. They are microscopic, but they are not doing the brain any good. They are a sign of a disease process.

I should mention that "plaque" is a generic word that refers to any sort of unwanted deposit. So you could have plaque on your teeth, plaques clogging your arteries, or microscopic plaques in your brain. They have nothing in common, except that the same word is used in each case.

Scientists have teased these beta-amyloid plaques apart to see what is in them. After feverish research, we now have a good picture of what they are made of. What is actually inside those plaques is surprising. As we'll see in the next chapter, we can put this finding to use, starting today, to work toward preventing the buildup of these plaques in the first place.

Aside from the beta-amyloid plaques that lie between the brain cells, there is also something wrong *inside* the brain cells themselves. They contain what look like tangled balls of yarn.

Normally your brain cells have microscopic tubes—which scientists call *microtubules*—that maintain the cell's structure and help it to transport various things from place to place within the cell. To stabilize these microtubules, your cells use *tau* proteins (*tau* is just the Greek letter that is the equivalent of our letter "T"). And it's those *tau* proteins that are balled up in what neurologists call *neurofibrillary tangles*.

In 1906, German physician Alois Alzheimer spotted these odd plaques and tangles in the brain of a patient who had died in her mid-fifties after suffering from memory loss and behavioral problems. Although Dr. Alzheimer dutifully reported the existence of plaques and tangles, he had no idea what had caused them, and for the past century, researchers have struggled to find out.

A person assaulted by Alzheimer's disease has also lost brain cells, along with many of the synapses between brain cells—the connections they need to communicate with each other.

So where is all this leading? Ultimately, many people with Alzheimer's disease die of pneumonia, often because the disease has affected their ability to swallow, and food particles end up in their lungs.

All of these problems are what we now aim to prevent.

Genetics of Alzheimer's Disease

Genes play a role in Alzheimer's disease. Chromosomes 21, 14, and 1 hold genes that produce proteins (called *beta-amyloid precursor protein*, *presenilin 1*, and *presenilin 2*) that are involved in making the beta-amyloid that ends up in plaques. Mutations in these genes cause aggressive forms of Alzheimer's disease that can strike when people are just in their thirties, forties, or fifties.

Fortunately, these cases are rare. For the vast majority of people, the effect of genes is weaker.

The best-known genetic contributor is a gene called APOE. Located on chromosome 19, it holds the instructions for producing a protein called *apolipoprotein E* (which scientists abbreviate with small letters as *apoE*, to differentiate it from the gene). ApoE's job is to help carry fat and cholesterol from place to place. It also repairs brain cells and builds connections from one neuron to another.

Here is what counts: There are three different common versions (alleles) for the APOE gene, called e2, e3, and e4. The e4 variant is the one that has raised concerns about Alzheimer's risk. Compared with people who got the e3 allele from both parents,

What Genes Mean

Each of your genes is made of two *alleles*—one from your mother and one from your father. For example, your mother might have given you an allele for brown hair, while your father might have given you an allele for blond hair. Your genetic makeup—and, in this case, your hair color—depends on the combination of alleles that you received.

For Alzheimer's disease, the APOE gene is important. The three common alleles are:

e2: Reduced risk of Alzheimer's disease but increased risk of rare cholesterol problems and cardiovascular disease
e3: No increased Alzheimer's risk
e4: Increased risk of Alzheimer's disease, especially if the allele came from both parents

those who inherit the e4 allele from one parent have about three times the risk of developing Alzheimer's disease. People who get the e4 allele from both parents have ten to fifteen times the risk.[3,4]

People with the e2 allele have less Alzheimer's risk. But e2 has problems of its own, causing a higher risk of rare cholesterol problems and cardiovascular disease.

It is important to understand that genes work in many different ways. Certainly, some genes are dictators—the genes for hair or eye color, for example. If they call for you to have blond hair or brown eyes, that's it. Those dictatorial genes won't take no for an answer.

But the genes for Alzheimer's disease are more like committees. They don't give orders; they make suggestions. And research suggests that changes in diet and lifestyle—the steps you will read about shortly—can keep those genes from expressing themselves. Like dry seeds on the desert floor, they simply lie dormant. If you don't water them, they'll never sprout.

Should You Get Tested?

Doctors can check to see which APOE alleles you are carrying, using a simple blood test. So, should you get tested? Some people are eager to know as much as possible about themselves and find that genetic tests help them put their risks into perspective. On the other hand, there is nothing you can do to change your genes. And just as having an e4 allele does not guarantee that you will get Alzheimer's disease, having e2 or e3 alleles does not guarantee that you will not. Regardless of your genetics, you will want to follow the steps in the chapters that follow.

So even though the e4 allele is linked to increased risk of Alzheimer's disease, some people who have the e4 allele—even from both parents—never get the disease. And at least one-third of Alzheimer's patients do not have the e4 allele. Research suggests that food and lifestyle choices can help protect you, whatever genetic hand you've been dealt.

Alzheimer's is not the only neurodegenerative condition. Here are other common types:

Vascular Dementia

The blood vessels of the brain can be gradually damaged and narrowed. In the process, they no longer give the brain the oxygen it needs. Sometimes the narrowing is very much like that which occurs in the arteries to the heart. At these narrowed spots, blood clots can form, plugging the artery like a cork in a bottle. Clots and debris can also break free, passing downstream and plugging smaller blood vessels farther along. Sometimes arteries actually break open, leaking blood into the brain tissue.

When a loss of blood flow kills off brain cells, doctors diagnose a stroke (which they will call an *infarct*), and the result can be weakness or paralysis, as well as cognitive problems. Sometimes small, imperceptible strokes add up in what is called *multi-infarct dementia*.

In other cases, the problem is more diffuse, with gradual damage along the walls of the small vessels in the brain, disrupting blood flow to the brain.

Brain imaging techniques often allow doctors to see small strokes and loss of blood flow. These scans look different from those in Alzheimer's disease, where imaging would be likely to show brain shrinkage, especially in the hippocampus and parts of the cortex. Not uncommonly, vascular dementia and

Alzheimer's disease occur in the same person, so the symptoms and brain imaging findings will reflect both.

The good news is that vascular dementia is, to a large degree, preventable. By making food choices that reduce your blood pressure and cholesterol level, avoiding smoking, and getting plenty of exercise, you'll have more power to keep your arteries healthy.

Stroke

Stroke is a common cause of dementia, often accompanied by physical weakness. Here is what you need to know:

Even though it makes up only about 2 percent of your body, your brain gets a good 20 percent of your blood supply, and for good reason. There are more cells in your brain than there are lightbulbs in Las Vegas (that is, 100 billion neurons and 10 times that many *glial* cells supporting them), and you need a steady stream of oxygen and nutrients to power them all. *A failure in the blood supply to the brain can result in stroke, and stroke is one of the leading causes of memory loss.*

To make sure your brain's blood supply doesn't fail, your heart uses not one but two separate sets of arteries. The *carotid* arteries are in the front of your neck, one on the left and the other on the right. If you gently place a finger just to the side of your windpipe, you'll feel a carotid artery beating. A second set, called the *vertebral* arteries, is deeper in the neck, passing up along the spine. This quartet of arteries join together at the base of the brain, so if one artery is blocked or damaged, blood can shuttle in from another.

From there, branches extend to the front of your brain, where your thoughts take shape and you plan your movements. Other branches reach the back of your brain, where vision is processed. Near the center of the brain is the limbic system, where brain cells cook up emotions. A dense network of nerves connects and coordinates all these regions. With a good blood supply, these structures will last a lifetime.

As well designed as the system is, things go wrong surprisingly often. As we saw earlier, arteries can become narrowed, clots can form, and bits of clot can end up plugging small arteries deep inside the brain.

A clot may also originate in the heart. In a condition called *atrial fibrillation,* an erratic heartbeat leads to pooling of blood within the heart, forming clots that can break away and flow upward toward the brain. The result is a stroke—or, in medical terms, a *cerebrovascular accident*—meaning that part of the brain has died.

Blood vessels can also break open. If an artery bursts in the brain, blood spills into the brain tissue, like water spraying out of a nick in a fire hose. The resulting pressure can kill brain cells.

While Alzheimer's disease begins very gradually, a stroke is not usually so subtle. If you are lucky, the affected area will be tiny, so symptoms are imperceptible. But small strokes can add up. Strokes that are too small to show up on brain scans occur surprisingly often and, collectively, they can affect a broad range

When Should You Worry?

When a stroke occurs, quick treatment is *essential*. For strokes caused by clots, clot-dissolving drugs often help if used within the first few hours. For hemorrhagic stroke, surgery may be necessary to remove accumulated blood or repair damaged blood vessels.

Unfortunately, the first signs of a stroke can be so vague that you are not sure whether to take them seriously. A hemorrhagic stroke, for example, can start with a headache. But headaches

(continued)

have many causes, of course. The signs that a headache may be caused by bleeding into the brain include sudden onset, severe pain, occurrence while lying down, worsening with movement and straining, such as coughing, or awakening you from sleep.

Here are other signs to look out for. Note that for the first day or so, symptoms can come and go.

- Change in alertness
- Seizure
- Confusion, memory loss, or trouble understanding others
- Changes in senses (numbness, tingling, or changes in vision, hearing, or taste)
- Weakness, clumsiness, or loss of balance
- Difficulty swallowing
- Difficulty reading or writing
- Dizziness or vertigo
- Loss of bladder or bowel control
- Sudden personality change

Often changes in strength or sensation are on just one side of the body.

of brain functions.[5] Often a single large stroke can wipe out a large part of the brain in one go. It can occur out of the blue, with paralysis, speech difficulties, and confusion that can be very sudden and frightening.

Doctors can often tell where a stroke has occurred based on the symptoms. Because the nerves cross over from one side of the body to the other, a stroke on one side of the brain manifests as weakness on the opposite side. The parts of the brain that control speech are mainly on the left. Vision is in the back.

Diagnosing a stroke: When doctors suspect a stroke, they conduct a careful neurological examination that checks your strength, senses (including vision), reflexes, and ability to speak and understand. They will also check your blood pressure and may listen for a "bruit" (pronounced *BROO-ee*, the French word for "noise") in your neck—a sound produced by disturbed blood flow in a carotid artery.

Brain imaging methods, including CT (computed tomography) and MRI (magnetic resonance imaging), allow doctors to see abnormalities within the brain. Doctors will also check the health of your heart and the arteries to the brain and run blood tests that detect clotting abnormalities, diabetes, and cholesterol problems. If your doctor suspects bleeding, he or she may do a spinal tap.

Doctors run through a checklist of medical conditions that could be mistaken for a stroke: migraine, low or high blood sugar, a seizure, an infection, multiple sclerosis, or a brain tumor.

The good news about strokes is that the brain can recover, at least to a degree. Even so, it is not an easy process by any means. Stroke recovery is often only partial, and it is often complicated by medical problems, including depression, as the brain seemingly shuts down other functions in order to focus on healing.

The steps outlined in the next several chapters will give you new power for controlling your weight, blood pressure, blood sugar, and cholesterol, which, in turn, will cut your risk of stroke.

Dementia with Lewy Bodies

This common cause of dementia is marked by the presence of Lewy bodies, which are clumps of proteins inside brain cells. They are named for Friedrich Lewy, the researcher who discovered them in the early 1900s.

Dr. Lewy found these abnormalities in patients with Parkinson's disease, the movement disorder made well-known by Muhammad Ali and Michael J. Fox, and, in recent years, researchers have shown that dementia with Lewy bodies and Parkinson's disease are related. Both conditions present problems with movement and mental function.

To separate dementia with Lewy bodies from Alzheimer's disease, doctors look for three main findings:

- Changes in alertness (An affected person may be alert at times, then become drowsy or stare off into space for prolonged periods.)
- Visual hallucinations
- Disordered movements

Brain scans are used as well, and may help to differentiate dementia with Lewy bodies from vascular dementia or Alzheimer's disease. A special type of brain imaging, called SPECT, is sometimes used to show changes in dopamine activity.

Frontotemporal Dementia

This is a group of disorders that mainly affect the frontal and temporal lobes of the brain. Most cases strike early—affecting people in their fifties or sixties—and many appear to have a genetic basis.

The main problems occur with language and behavior. You could have trouble finding words, speaking, or understanding what others are saying. Behavior can become uninhibited and inappropriate, or sometimes just listless and lethargic. Brain scanning methods show shrinkage and reduced activity in the affected areas.

Cognitive problems can also be a complication of Huntington's disease or Creutzfeldt-Jakob disease, as well as any of the common medical conditions outlined in chapter 8.

Those are the threats we need to be aware of. Some of them—

most notably Alzheimer's disease and stroke—are strongly linked to choices we make.

Building Your Shield

By now, you are probably frightened, considering all the things that can go wrong. Well, this is the time for action. In the next several chapters, we will draw on scientific research to build a powerful shield to protect your brain.

We will start with a look at foods—foods that help us and other foods that we will want to steer clear of. We will also turn our attention to exercises—mental and physical—that can strengthen the brain. We will see how to give your memory banks the rest they need and how to protect your brain from the surprising array of assaults that can take away your edge.

If Frances stayed reasonably clear all her life, while her sister Mary Lou developed more serious memory problems, what made the difference? Could it be that Frances ate considerably more healthfully? Or could it be the fact that she was a much more avid reader? Or maybe it was the exercise program she went to after work? Or perhaps it was all of these things.

In the following chapters, we will see exactly how to protect your memory. Here's how we'll proceed:

• First, I want you to understand a few basics of how foods affect brain function. It is easy but important. Certain food components are toxic to the brain, and you are almost certainly exposed to many of them now. I want to point them out to you so you can protect yourself. And there are protective nutrients, too—critically important natural compounds, and I'll show you where to find them. So please take your time and go through these pages carefully.

• Second, we will want to reinforce your brain synapses with cognitive exercises that are simple and fun. As you will see, this takes very little time, but the results can be quite striking. Then we will pump up blood flow to your brain using an individualized program of physical conditioning. It is extremely easy, and you can build up to however challenging a level you might like. The result can be measurable changes in brain structure.

• Third, it is critical to restore your brain's ability to integrate memories and to retrieve them. That means using sleep for all it's worth—and many people have an abysmal night's sleep for months or years on end. I will show you how to take an inventory of your sleep habits and correct them if you need to. It also means looking at medications and medical conditions that cause brain cells to misfire. We will go through them in an easy but systematic way.

I hope you will explore the menus and recipes in this book and have fun with them. If you are surprised that healthful recipes could seem so delicious, the fact is that two top chefs designed them that way. Together, we aim to seduce your taste buds so you cannot help but fall into good health.

Over the short run, you'll find that you are not only protecting your brain. You're also enhancing your health. Over the long run, you'll be less and less likely to succumb to the physical problems that others face.

Healthful eating also opens the doors to a world of delights you had never anticipated. So by using the power of food, adding brain-strengthening exercises, and understanding how medicines and medical conditions interact with brain function, you will have a powerful program for conquering memory problems and being at your best.

So what are we waiting for? Let's jump in!

Step I

PUT POWER FOODS TO WORK

Within the gray matter that makes up the outer layer of the brain are the billions of brain cells that allow you to think, speak, move, anticipate the future, and manage your day-to-day life. They link with each other via billions upon billions of synaptic connections and send even more links to other parts of the brain, to the muscles, and to your sense organs.

If you have memory problems, it is a sign that these connections are not working properly. Perhaps the brain cells are not getting the nutrients they need. Maybe they are momentarily misfiring, due to a side effect of some medication. Some connections may be broken, or perhaps the brain cells themselves are no longer there at all.

Researchers have worked long and hard to track down the causes of memory problems so we can take steps to prevent them. As we have seen, there are three key steps for protecting your memory.

We'll begin by zeroing in on what you're eating. First, certain metals can be toxic to the brain and have turned up in examinations of brain tissue from people with Alzheimer's. In the following chapter, we will see where they are coming from and how you can protect yourself. You may be shocked to learn where they are hiding. Then, in the next two chapters, we will look at the role of fats—some are distinctly harmful to the brain, surprisingly enough, while others are actually helpful—and at common vitamins that are essential for protecting the brain. It is important to know where to find them and how to put them to work.

CHAPTER 2

Foods That Shield You from Toxic Metals

The Beatles made an enormous splash in Liverpool. But as big as they were, there was one commodity that was much bigger and much more controversial.

Liverpool is a port city. So ships come and go, carrying coal, timber, grains, steel, crude oil, and endless other commodities. Loaded onto ships leaving Liverpool in the eighteenth century was the most controversial product in English history.

In their holds were bars of copper—that ordinary reddish metal that makes a pot or pan look so shiny and bright. Copper looks innocent enough. But it was the currency of the British slave trade.

The ships sailed from Liverpool to West Africa, where copper and brassware were exchanged for slaves who were then carried across the Atlantic to the Americas. There the human cargo was off-loaded, and rum and sugar from slave plantations were carried back to Britain. This triangular trade route from Britain to Africa to the Americas and back was fueled by copper from Liverpool. It was what African slaveholders wanted.

Copper also kept the ships afloat. Sailing around the North Atlantic, wooden ships worked out well. But as slave ships entered the Caribbean, they encountered a tiny mollusk, called *Teredo navalis,* which feeds on wood. Or, more accurately, these mollusks have a special organ that carries a bacterium that digests cellulose, dissolving the hulls of ships. A few too many mollusks and your ship is on the ocean bottom.

The answer was to sheathe the hulls in copper. Copper kept the mollusks out, the hulls intact, and the slave ships sailing.

Many Britons called for an end to the slave trade. But copper merchants protested vigorously. They were not getting rich selling pots and pans in Lancashire. The slave trade was the market they wanted to protect. Finally, in 1807, public sentiment turned, and it became illegal for British subjects to traffic in slaves. In 1833, slavery was abolished in all British colonies.

Metals in the Brain

Metals always seem to come in the form of double-edged swords. Lead gave us pipes for plumbing, but it has also poisoned countless children. Mercury gave us thermometers and electrical switches, but it also caused birth defects. Metals build bridges and locomotives, and also bullets, prison cells, and hand grenades.

Metals are a double-edged sword within the human brain, too. In the last chapter, we saw that researchers have found *plaques* and *tangles* within the brains of people with Alzheimer's disease. If you were to analyze a typical plaque—one of the small deposits that are found among the brain cells—you would discover that much of it consists of *beta-amyloid* protein. But there is something else there, too. Teasing the plaques apart, researchers have found traces of copper. They have found other metals, too, particularly iron and zinc, and perhaps others, as well.[1]

All three of these metals are needed by the body—copper for building enzymes, iron for blood cells, and zinc for nerve transmission, among many other functions. You get them in the foods you eat. But it turns out that if you get too much of any of them, they can damage your brain cells. The difference between a safe amount and a toxic amount is surprisingly small. And that is exactly the problem.

Iron and copper are unstable. Just pour a little water into a cast-iron pan and let it sit for a bit. The rust you see is oxidation. Copper oxidizes, too, which is why a bright shiny penny soon darkens, sometimes combining with other elements and turning green.

Pretty colors, yes. What is not so pretty is when these chemical reactions happen inside your body. That's when iron and copper spark the production of *free radicals*—highly unstable and destructive oxygen molecules that can damage your brain cells and accelerate the aging process.[2] In a nutshell, iron and copper cause free radicals to form, and those free radicals are like torpedoes attacking your cells.

So, am I saying that memory problems might be caused by ordinary metals like copper, iron, and zinc? To help answer that question, let me take you to Rome, where a research team studied sixty-four women.[3] All were over age fifty but perfectly healthy. The researchers drew blood samples to measure copper in their blood and then gave them a variety of tests to check their memory, reasoning, language comprehension, and ability to concentrate.

Now, overall the women did just fine. None had any major

impairment. But some did noticeably better than others on one test or another. And *those who had the least mental difficulties turned out to be those with lower levels of copper in their blood.* They had adequate copper for the body's needs but were free of excesses, and that apparently did them a big favor. The difference was especially noticeable on tests that required focused attention.

A study of sixty-four women is not especially large. So let's next drop in on a research team at the University of California at San Diego that evaluated a much larger group, this one consisting of 1,451 people in Southern California.[4] They found much the same thing. People who had lower copper levels in their blood were mentally clearer compared with those with excessive copper. They had fewer problems with short-term and long-term memory. And the same held true for iron. People with less iron in their blood had fewer memory problems.

So even though both iron and copper are essential in tiny amounts, having too much of either one in your bloodstream seems to spell trouble.

If this sounds surprising, it did not entirely surprise the researchers. Every medical student knows that copper is potentially toxic. Your body uses tiny amounts of it in enzymes for various functions, but the amount you need is extremely small. If you get too much of this unstable metal, it can oxidize and encourage free radicals to form. In fact, the only thing that stops copper from destroying your health early in life is that your liver filters much of it out of your blood and eliminates it. In a rare genetic condition called Wilson's disease, the liver is unable to eliminate copper normally. As copper builds up in the body tissues, it damages the central nervous system and causes all manner of other problems.

Similarly, excess iron has long been known to cause potentially serious health problems. More on iron in a minute. But first, let's deal with copper and understand what it is doing to our brains.

I should tell you that copper may contribute to much more serious problems than the minor variations in memory and cognition seen in the Rome and San Diego studies. Starting in 1993, a research team from Rush University Medical Center went door-to-door in three Chicago neighborhoods, aiming to track down the causes of health problems that occur as we age. They invited 6,158 people to join the Chicago Health and Aging Project, and eventually another 3,000 joined in, as well.

The researchers carefully recorded what the volunteers ate. Like people everywhere, some were health conscious, while others were not so particular. The research team then kept in touch with everyone over the years to see who stayed well and who did not—who kept their mental clarity and who had memory problems. They then looked to see if any part of the diet could have predicted who might fall prey to memory loss.

Now, many of the participants got adequate copper in their diets, without excesses. As the years went by, they generally did well on the cognitive tests the researchers gave them. But other participants got quite a bit more of it. Needless to say, none of them were worrying about anything so insignificant as copper. Who would even have known it was in foods, anyway? But as time went on, a particular combination seemed to be especially harmful. Those whose diets included fair amounts of copper along with certain "bad" fats—the fats found in animal products and snack foods—showed a loss of mental function that was the equivalent of *an extra nineteen years of aging.*[5] It appears that "bad" fats team up with copper to attack the brain. These fats actually assault the brain in many ways, as we'll see in the next chapter.

The difference in copper intake between those who generally did well and those who did not was surprisingly small. Here are the numbers: For comparison, a penny weighs 2,500 milligrams. The people in the Chicago study who generally avoided cognitive problems got around 1 milligram of copper per day. Those who did not do so well averaged around 3 milligrams per day (2.75 milligrams, to be exact). One milligram, three milligrams—what's the difference? you might be asking. That is still just a tiny speck of copper. But it turned out to be more than enough to cause serious problems. As we will see shortly, the foods that deliver this innocent-looking, bright, shiny metal are right under our noses, and it damages the brain enough to interfere with attention, learning, and memory—and perhaps even cause Alzheimer's disease. Or so research seems to show.

Copper and Cognitive Loss

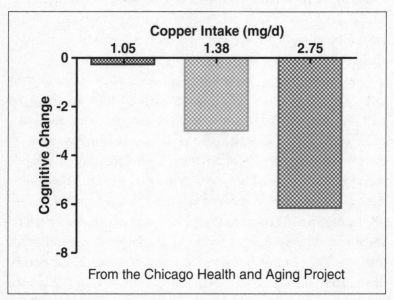

People in the Chicago Health and Aging Project who got the most copper in their diets—averaging 2.75 milligrams per day—along with fatty diets lost much more cognitive function as time went on compared with people who had less copper in their diets.

Copper and Genes

Researchers have found a surprising link between copper and the APOE e4 allele—that is, the gene linked to Alzheimer's risk. As you'll recall, the proteins made by the APOE e2 and APOE e3 alleles are not associated with increased Alzheimer's risk. It turns out that these two "safer" genes make proteins that *bind copper.* They keep it out of harm's way. The protein produced by APOE e4 does not do that. As far as APOE e4 is concerned, you are on your own. It does nothing to protect you from copper and the shower of free radicals it causes.[6]

Iron, Zinc, and Rusty Brain Cells

Copper is not the only problem. Iron builds up in the body in a condition called *hemochromatosis,* causing fatigue, weakness, and pain, and ultimately leading to heart disease, diabetes, liver damage, arthritis, and many other problems.

In the Netherlands, researchers measured iron levels in healthy research volunteers using simple blood tests. Naturally, they varied a bit in their iron levels; some were lower and others were higher. The research team then tested everyone's memory, reaction speed, and other cognitive abilities. And the results were remarkably similar to the findings with copper. Those who were slowest on cognitive tests were those who had the most iron in their blood.[7]

Your body packs iron into hemoglobin, the iron-containing protein that gives your red blood cells their color and allows them to carry oxygen. In 2009, a group of researchers checked hemoglobin levels in a large group of older men and women. Those whose hemoglobin levels were in the healthy range did well on cognitive tests. But some people were not in this range.

Some were anemic. They had low hemoglobin levels, and they did not perform well on cognitive tests. And other people were in the opposite situation—they had unusually *high* hemoglobin levels. They did poorly, too. Specifically, they had problems with verbal memory (e.g., recalling words) and perception.[8]

Following these people for the next three years, those whose hemoglobin levels were in the healthy range tended to retain their mental clarity. Those who were too low or too high in hemoglobin showed more rapid cognitive decline. People with high hemoglobin levels were more than three times more likely to develop Alzheimer's disease compared with those who were in the healthy hemoglobin range.[9] The safest hemoglobin level was around 13.7 grams per deciliter. Going very far above or below that level was linked to problems with brain function as the years went by.

Keep in mind that in these studies hemoglobin was a rough indicator of how much iron people had in their bodies. While you need some iron, it is dangerous to get too much.

Zinc is similar in that your body needs a tiny amount. In fact, your brain cells use zinc to communicate with each other.[10,11] But in overdose, zinc can be potentially toxic.

So let's return to the question at hand. Could it be that memory problems are caused by getting too much of these seemingly ordinary metals—copper, iron, and zinc? While research is still very active, here's the picture that is emerging:

All three metals—copper, iron, and zinc—are clearly present in the beta-amyloid plaques of Alzheimer's disease. The first two—copper and iron—appear to spark the production of free radicals that can damage brain cells.[2,12] Zinc's contribution appears to be different. It seems to encourage beta-amyloid proteins to clump together to form plaques.[10,11] Iron and copper appear to promote clumping, too, but zinc seems to be much more aggressive in this regard.[1]

So it may be that these metals work together, encouraging plaques to form and generating free radicals that attack brain cells. And the problems appear to start early in life, as mild memory problems that pass for everyday forgetfulness, as well as in mild cognitive impairment that for many people is a step toward Alzheimer's disease.

Where Are Metals Coming From?

By now, you are no doubt visualizing toxic metals picking off your brain cells one by one. Well, where are these metals coming from?

Let's start in your kitchen. What's under your sink? Copper plumbing has been popular since the 1930s. As copper pipes and brass fittings corrode, copper leaches into drinking water.[13]

Is there a cast-iron pan on your stove? Iron cookware contributes a significant amount of iron to foods. While that may be beneficial for a young woman with monthly iron losses through menstruation, most other people are more likely to be iron-overloaded than iron-deficient.

Next, take a look in your kitchen cupboard. Do you keep a bottle of multiple vitamins? A One A Day Men's Health Formula multivitamin has 2 milligrams of copper—more than twice the RDA—in a single pill. It exceeds the RDA for zinc, too. In fact, if you take a look at most any vitamin-mineral supplement, you'll find copper, zinc, and sometimes iron.

So many of us imagine we are doing a smart thing by taking a daily multiple vitamin, and we are, in many ways. It's an excellent source of vitamin B_{12} and vitamin D, both of which are important for health. But the metals that are often added are mostly unnecessary, because *you are already getting them in foods.* A better choice is a supplement containing vitamins only, without the added copper, zinc, iron, or other minerals. Or you could choose a B-complex tablet, which limits itself to just B vitamins. We will cover vitamins in more detail in chapter 4.

In the 1950s, television commercials pushed Geritol as the answer to "iron-poor tired blood." The tonic had "twice the iron in a whole pound of calf's liver." Doctors promoted iron supplements as an energy booster, too, on the theory that sluggishness was a sign of anemia. Not that they worked very well; fatigue has many causes, and iron deficiency is nowhere near the top of the list.

Take a look at your breakfast cereal. No doubt the food scientists at General Mills imagined you wanted all the iron and zinc they've added to a box of Total—a full day's supply of each in every serving. But you do not need these added metals, and you are better off without them. Many other breakfast cereals are similar, giving you too much of a good thing. I have asked General Mills and the other major cereal manufacturers to limit their supplementation to vitamins and to leave out minerals, which most customers get plenty of already.

So plumbing, cookware, supplement pills, and fortified cereals—these all contribute to an overdose of metals that will do your brain no good. But none of these are the biggest source.

Metals in Common Foods

To see the mother lode of metal, stop into any coffee shop in Chicago and order liver and onions. No, don't eat it. Send it to a laboratory. You would be amazed at what you find.

For comparison, the recommended dietary allowance for

copper is 0.9 milligram, as we saw above. A typical serving of liver (about 3½ ounces) has *more than 14 milligrams* of copper. It also has 7 milligrams of iron and 5 milligrams of zinc, not to mention nearly 400 milligrams of cholesterol.

Now, many people avoid liver because it harbors such an enormous load of cholesterol, among other problems. But they are busily chowing down on beef and other meats. Growing up in North Dakota, I certainly did, and so did my parents and most of the people we knew. Unbeknownst to us, meat-heavy diets are a major source of excess metals.

This is, in fact, a key difference between my North Dakota diet on the one hand, and a plant-based diet on the other. Take iron for starters. Green vegetables and beans contain iron. But it is in a special form called *nonheme iron,* which the body is able to regulate. That is, nonheme iron is more absorbable if you are low in iron and less absorbable if you already have plenty of iron in your body. That is an amazing feature, if you think about it. The amount of iron in a leaf of spinach or a sprig of broccoli does not change from minute to minute. But how much of it your body absorbs does change depending on how much you need. If you happened to have plenty of iron in your blood already, your body is able to turn down its absorption of the nonheme iron in green vegetables. And if you're running low, your body pulls more of the vegetable's iron into your bloodstream.

Meats contain some of this kind of iron. But they also contain a great deal of what is called *heme* iron. And heme iron is harder for your body to regulate. Even if you have plenty of iron in your body already, heme iron is still very absorbable compared to nonheme iron. It is like an uninvited guest just barging in on your party. It can tip you into iron overload.

Cows get iron from grass and concentrate it in blood cells and muscle tissue. If we eat meat, we ingest the concentrated iron that animals have stored, and it ends up being more than we need. If instead we were to eat plants directly, we would get the iron we need, without much risk of an overdose.

We're like the big fish in the ocean. A little fish ingests a bit of mercury from pollutants in the water. A bigger fish then eats the little one and gets all the mercury in the smaller fish's body. In turn, this fish is swallowed by an even bigger one, who now gets all the mercury that has been accumulating up the food chain. And that's us. We are the big fish in the ocean, so to speak, ingesting whatever the animals we eat have accumulated during their lives.

It is a good idea to step out of the food chain and take advantage of the nutrition that plants bring us directly. In research studies, we have done exactly that. That is, we have asked people to skip meat and other animal products. So breakfast might be blueberry pancakes or old-fashioned oatmeal topped with sliced bananas. Lunch might be lentil soup with crusty bread, a bean burrito with Spanish rice, a veggie burger, or a spinach salad. Dinner could be a vegetable stir-fry, mushroom Stroganoff with steamed broccoli, or angel-hair pasta topped with artichoke hearts, seared oyster mushrooms, and Roma tomatoes. As we add up the amount of iron in the foods they have chosen, it is usually the same or slightly more than when they were eating meat. However, as these foods pass their lips, their digestive tract has the surprising ability to decide how much or how little iron it needs to absorb. If they have a lot of iron on board already, their iron absorption is automatically reduced. If they need iron, their iron absorption is increased. And that is possible because the iron they are getting is nonheme iron. As a rule, it gives you what you need without the excess.

Plant-based diets also help you avoid the overdose of zinc and copper. There are adequate amounts of these minerals in vegetables, beans, and whole grains. In fact, there may be more copper in these foods than in meats. But if you were to do blood tests on people who avoid meat, you would find that they are slightly lower in iron, copper, and zinc, which is a good thing.[14,15] The reasons for this are not entirely clear. Aside from your body's ability to shut out nonheme iron, there is a natural substance called *phytic acid* in many plants that tends to limit copper and zinc absorption.[14,15]

Years ago, all this made nutritionists nervous. After all, we need traces of each of these metals, and many nutrition experts cautioned vegetarians to take extra care to get plenty of iron and zinc. And they reassured meat eaters that they had nothing to worry about.[16]

Today things have turned around. Nutrition researchers have been struck by the observation that people following plant-based diets tend to keep their iron levels in the healthy range. They are no more likely than meat eaters to dip into anemia, but they are much *less* likely to accumulate excess iron.[14] Vegetarians tend to do fine with copper and zinc, too.

Let me emphasize that it is indeed important to get each of these metals in foods. You need them and do not want to run low. But it is just as important to avoid poisoning yourself with excessive amounts. Getting nutrition from plant sources is the easiest way to stay in the healthy zone.

Growing up in North Dakota, vegetables and beans were not exactly our strong suit. Meat was at the center of our plates 365 days a year. At the time we thought we were doing well. Today we know better.

How Much Do You Really Need?

Here are the recommended daily allowances, showing how much copper, iron, and zinc your body needs. It is important to include these minerals in your diet, but it is also important to avoid excesses.

Copper: 0.9 milligram per day for men and women. Healthful sources include beans, green leafy vegetables, nuts, whole grains, and mushrooms.

Iron: 8 milligrams per day for adult men and for women over fifty; 18 milligrams for women between nineteen and fifty. Healthful sources include green leafy vegetables, beans, whole grains, and dried fruits.

Zinc: 11 milligrams per day for men, 8 milligrams per day for women. Healthful sources include oatmeal, whole-grain bread, brown rice, peanuts, beans, nuts, peas, and sesame seeds.

Does Aluminum Harm the Brain?

In the world of Alzheimer's research, the most hotly debated metal is not any of the ones we've discussed so far. It is aluminum.

In the 1970s, researchers analyzed the brains of people who had died of various causes. In people who had not developed Alzheimer's disease, researchers found very little aluminum. But many of those who had had Alzheimer's had quite a bit of aluminum in their brains—in one case as much as 107 micrograms of aluminum per gram of brain tissue.[17,18] Yes, it's the same stuff that is in soda cans and aluminum foil, and particles of it were inside their brains.

What was it doing there? Our nutritional requirement for aluminum is exactly zero. It has no role in brain function at all, nor does it play a part in any other aspect of human biology.

For many years, public health officials have known that large doses of aluminum are harmful. People exposed to unusually large amounts in the workplace or who have received aluminum in renal dialysis solutions have sometimes developed serious brain damage and have needed a treatment called *chelation* to remove the metal from their bodies.

As a result of these studies, aluminum became a suspect in the Alzheimer's epidemic.[19,20] Researchers began to debate whether the traces of aluminum we might be exposed to from day to day—in pots and pans or in food additives—could put us at risk.

To this day, the question has not been settled. Some disconcerting evidence came from British researchers who measured aluminum in drinking water. Normally there is almost no aluminum in water as it arrives from wells or streams. But at municipal water purification plants, a process called *flocculation* introduces aluminum as a way of removing suspended particles. In turn, traces of aluminum stay in the water, and they flow from your tap when you fill your drinking glass.

Looking at the tap water in eighty-eight county districts in the UK, the researchers found that the aluminum content varied greatly. In some it exceeded 0.11 milligram per liter. In others it was less than one-tenth that amount. They then looked at Alzheimer's cases and found they were 50 percent more frequent in the high-aluminum counties.[21]

A French study found much the same result.[22] In a group of 1,925 people, those with more aluminum in their drinking water had a faster cognitive decline and were more likely to be diagnosed with Alzheimer's disease.

Canadian studies added to the accumulating evidence. A high incidence of Alzheimer's disease in a small part of Newfoundland was hard to explain, except that the local drinking water had particularly high levels of aluminum.[23] A study in

Quebec linked aluminum in drinking water to a nearly threefold increased risk of Alzheimer's disease.[24] A study in Newcastle, UK, seemed to disprove the hypothesis, finding no strong relationship between aluminum and Alzheimer's,[25,26] until it became clear that there just was not as much aluminum in the water there compared with areas where the link had been found.[27]

Since then, researchers have debated whether aluminum is a problem or not.[19,28] Many feel the evidence indicting aluminum is not particularly strong. The Alzheimer's Association calls the aluminum-Alzheimer's link a "myth" and had this to say on its website:

> During the 1960s and 1970s, aluminum emerged as a possible suspect in Alzheimer's. This suspicion led to concern about exposure to aluminum through everyday sources such as pots and pans, beverage cans, antacids and antiperspirants. Since then, studies have failed to confirm any role for aluminum in causing Alzheimer's. Experts today focus on other areas of research, and few believe that everyday sources of aluminum pose any threat.[29]

Many authorities agree with this viewpoint. They feel that small amounts of aluminum do little harm and that your kidneys ought to be able to eliminate the incidental traces you might ingest in drinking water and other day-to-day exposures. Perhaps the aluminum deposits found in Alzheimer's patients' brains are just a sign that an already-diseased brain can no longer keep toxins out.

However, others have felt the evidence against aluminum is too strong to ignore,[19] and in 2011 a group of Alzheimer's researchers published the following comment in the *International Journal of Alzheimer's Disease*:

There is growing evidence for a link between aluminum and Alzheimer's disease, and between other metals and Alzheimer's disease. Nevertheless, because the precise mechanism of Alzheimer's disease pathogenesis remains unknown, this issue is controversial. However, it is widely accepted that aluminum is a recognized neurotoxin, and that it could cause cognitive deficiency and dementia when it enters the brain and may have various adverse effects on the central nervous system.[30]

So what are we to make of this? Is aluminum a problem or not? I suggest that you not feel a need to take a stand on this unresolved issue. There is no need to bet your brain one way or the other. Instead, it is prudent to simply err on the side of caution. Since you don't need aluminum, it makes sense to avoid it to the extent you can. You cannot avoid it all, but choosing aluminum-free products lets you steer clear of major exposures.

Aluminum turns up in a surprising range of products. At the University of Kentucky in Lexington, Robert Yokel, PhD, found large amounts of aluminum in many common foods—much more than British, French, or Canadian people were getting in their tap water.

How could that be? The U.S. Food and Drug Administration considers certain aluminum-containing food additives to be GRAS—"generally recognized as safe"—so food manufacturers are free to use them. Aluminum compounds serve as emulsifying agents in cheese, especially on frozen pizza. It is in common baking powders and the products prepared with them. It is in foil and in cookware, and, yes, your spaghetti sauce will pick up a substantial amount of aluminum from an aluminum pot. It is in soda cans, which can leach aluminum into the products they hold.[31]

Luckily, there are perfectly suitable alternatives for most every aluminum-containing product. Which leads us to how we can protect ourselves from toxic metals.

How to Shield Yourself

As I have mentioned, research on toxic metals in Alzheimer's disease is still very much in progress. But some things are clear: There is never any benefit from overdoing it with copper, iron, or zinc, and there is no need to ingest aluminum at all. Here are sensible steps you can put to work right now to protect yourself:

Check Your Foods

- Get your protein from plant sources rather than meats. Organ meats (such as liver) and shellfish (such as lobster and crab) are loaded with metals, not to mention cholesterol. And meats in general—not just liver—tend to deliver more iron and other metals than the body can safely handle. Beans and green leafy vegetables provide iron in a safer (nonheme) form that is more absorbable if you need iron and less absorbable if you have plenty of iron in your body already.

- Check the labels on processed foods. You already wanted to skip frozen pizza, because of all the fat and cholesterol in the cheese and meat toppings. Many brands also have aluminum in the cheese and/or crust, as you'll see on the labels. A good rule of thumb is that the simpler your foods, the more confidence you can have about what is in them. Everything in the produce aisle, for example, has just one ingredient.

- Choose aluminum-free baking powder. Aluminum-free brands are widely available. Unfortunately, restaurants are not likely to tell you what sort of baking powder they use, and their pancakes can contain substantial aluminum traces without your knowing it.

- Skip the single-serve creamers and salt packets. They often contain sodium aluminosilicate, an anticaking agent that keeps them pourable.[32]
- Check labels on pickle relish. Some contain aluminum.

Check Your Cookware and Containers

- Choose safe cookware. All kitchen stores sell cookware that is free of copper and iron on cooking surfaces. When using aluminum foil, keep it from touching any acidic foods.
- Avoid aluminum cans. Aluminum soda cans have a lining that is supposed to block the aluminum from ending up in the product, but it is not an entirely effective barrier. The longer the soda sits in the can, the more aluminum passes into it. Bottles may be safer, and quitting soda altogether is the best idea.

Check Your Cupboards

- Be careful in your choice of vitamin supplements. Most vitamin-mineral supplements marketed for older people now omit iron, but they typically do include copper and zinc. It makes sense to choose a supplement with vitamins only, omitting minerals.
- Use only aluminum-free antacids if you use antacids. Maalox gets its brand name from the *MA*gnesium and *AL*uminum hydr*OX*ide inside. It can easily deliver a thousand times more aluminum than you would get from a day's worth of foods. Aluminum is also found in Mylanta

and Gaviscon. But Tums, Rolaids, and many others do not contain aluminum; they are made with calcium carbonate instead. By the way, if you have an ulcer, the best treatment is an antibiotic, not an antacid. Ulcers are typically caused by the *Helicobacter pylori* bacteria, which can be eliminated with a brief antibiotic regimen.

- Read the labels on over-the-counter medicines. Some add aluminum as a coloring agent.

- Use a deodorant, not an antiperspirant. Common antiperspirants contain aluminum, which passes through the skin and into your bloodstream. Products labeled as *deodorants,* but not as *antiperspirants,* typically omit aluminum. Now, if you are nervous that avoiding aluminum-containing products would mean you are condemned to using natural deodorants that smell of patchouli and don't actually work, you will be glad to know that you can still access products from the same chemical conglomerates that make the aluminum-containing brands. If you read a few labels at the drugstore, you'll see. And you'll also find many aluminum-free natural brands, some of which do indeed work. Beware of those containing alum. That's simply an aluminum compound.

Check Your Beverages

- See how your tap water stacks up for safety, or use bottled springwater. The Environmental Protection Agency maintains water quality records that show the metal content in some US locales at its website, http://cfpub.epa .gov/safewater/ccr. If you are unsure about your tap water, bottled springwater may be a better choice. Some home water-filter units (such as reverse osmosis systems) effectively remove aluminum. If you have copper plumbing, use tap water for household uses but not for cooking or drinking.

- Minimize your use of tea. The tea plant (*Camellia sinensis*) draws minerals from the soil, and aluminum tends to concentrate in the leaves. The aluminum content in tea is less than in foods overall but still significant.

For Extra Credit

- Exercise helps you rid your body of excess iron. In chapter 6, we'll see how to get started.
- Surprising as it may sound, donating blood is the fastest way to eliminate excess stored iron. And you're giving it to someone who can actually use it.

What About Mercury?

By now you might be thinking, "Wait a minute! I've got mercury in my fillings! Could that be a problem, too?" I wish I had a definitive answer for you. There is no question that mercury can harm the brain, which is one of the reasons that health authorities have sounded the alarm about tuna and certain other fish for pregnant women and children. Some researchers have pointed out that mercury amalgam fillings increase the amount of mercury going to the brain by anywhere from twofold to tenfold.[33] Others have suggested a link with multiple sclerosis.[34] That said, there have been too few studies to make any solid conclusions. A large Minnesota study found no links between mercury amalgam fillings and Alzheimer's disease.[35]

My best guess is that it is prudent to replace existing mercury fillings with safer compounds and to avoid getting any new ones, but I do not expect that research studies will be able to settle this question in the foreseeable future.

The Bottom Line on Metals

The discovery that metals are hiding inside beta-amyloid plaques and the revelation that these metals might contribute to everything from everyday mental fuzziness to Alzheimer's disease were huge breakthroughs in medicine.

While research continues, you'll want to remember that you do need some copper, iron, and zinc, but all of these metals are toxic in excess. You don't need aluminum *at all*. Simple steps will help you avoid potentially risky exposures.

There is much, much more to protecting your memory and cognition. The next chapter deals with one of the most common and decisive issues in brain function—the fats that end up on our plates and in our bodies.

CHAPTER 3

Foods That Protect You from Harmful Fats and Cholesterol

The next clue comes not from a laboratory but from a garden, where a woman named Masu is working. She spent the morning cleaning her house, doing her chores, and tending her plants, and she is now picking lettuce, spinach, and green onions for her lunch. The fact that she turned 100 last year and is still active and in good health is not remarkable here. Many people in Okinawa live to a ripe old age. Her cousins are 105 and 106.

She has been through a lot over the years, including the hardships of World War II, when a quarter of the civilian population of Okinawa died and life for the rest was precarious. Foods from the family garden sustained them during those difficult times, just as they do today.

In the post–World War II period, Americans brought their own food preferences, and McDonald's and KFC eventually set up shop on the island. But Masu has never been to either one. Her number one staple is the sweet potato, with rice a close second. And she has plenty of greens, daikon radish, seaweed, and nigauri (or "bitter melon"), which is a bit like a cucumber. The occasional bit of fish or pork will find its way onto her plate, but these are not staples.

Her daughter moved to the United States and started a Japanese restaurant, where she serves many of the same foods that kept her family healthy. Have they heard of Alzheimer's disease in Okinawa? Yes, but it's not very common and, as her daughter told me, "that's only in really old people."

Masu didn't know it, but during World War II, sailing offshore on an American destroyer was a young military surgeon with whom she had quite a few things in common. Ellsworth Wareham, MD, was originally from Alberta, Canada. He moved to Loma Linda, California—about an hour east of Los Angeles—to go to medical school. After Pearl Harbor turned the world on its head, he found himself sailing past Okinawa. And what he was eating was very similar to a lunch Masu might have prepared for herself. As soon as hostilities ended, he pursued advanced studies in cardiothoracic surgery and eventually ended up back at Loma Linda University, serving as chief of cardiothoracic surgery.

The reason I am telling you all this is because just as there was something that set Okinawans apart from people in most other countries—their amazing health and longevity—there was something that set Ellsworth apart from other surgeons. He had energy they didn't have. When they retired, he kept going. Age sixty-five was just a number. As he reached seventy, seventy-five, and eighty years, he still donned his gloves and surgical gown and strode into the OR every day, just as he always had.

This can't go on forever, he told himself. So, arbitrarily, he decided that ninety-five ought to be the age when he would retire. And when that day finally arrived, that's what he did. Even though his colleagues tried to talk him into staying—they wanted his experience, steady hands, and clear mind at the operating table and even offered to pay his malpractice insurance premiums if he would stay—he figured it was time. He decided to hang up the scalpel—sort of. Today you'll find him operating on the bushes and trees on his two-acre lawn. At six feet tall and 172 pounds, he feels great. "I never have any aches or pains. I rarely have a cold or the flu."

So what is he eating? When he was growing up, Ellsworth's family raised cattle for beef and milk, and chickens for eggs. And he didn't particularly like the look of any of it.

"Looking after the animals, I found milk to be rather unhygienic, when you see where it comes from. The chickens were not too clean either, so I didn't care for their eggs. I had them once in a while, but not often. I never cared for meat or dairy products." And then, arriving in Loma Linda, his diet took another step. "I found out that I didn't need animal products *at all*. In fact, I was better off without them. And that was it. For the past four decades, I've pretty much avoided anything from animals."

Anywhere else, that might have been an odd choice. But Loma Linda is home to many Seventh-day Adventists, whose religious teachings put a huge premium on clean living. Tobacco, alcohol, and even caffeine are frowned on, and meat eating is discouraged, too. So skipping animal products entirely was not a particularly unusual choice.

Sailing by Okinawa, he would have loved a serving of Masu's sweet potatoes and vegetables. His own meals are just as simple. Fresh fruit and whole-grain cereal with soy milk for breakfast; baked beans, vegetables, corn on the cob, soy yogurt, and occasional faux "meats" later in the day; with almonds or peanuts as snacks. He enjoys his menu and the health and longevity it has brought him. He recalled a *Wall Street Journal* article that said that other than breast milk, all tastes are acquired. "In other words, your tastes adapt to what you eat. If you eat fatty, salty foods, those are the foods you'll crave. And if you break away from them, you'll come to enjoy healthier foods."

Lessons from the Blue Zones

Okinawa and Loma Linda are places where people enjoy surprisingly good health—including healthy brain function—well into advanced age. In 2005, these remarkable geographic "blue zones" were described by Dan Buettner in a *National Geographic* pictorial. Other "blue zones" include Sardinia, Italy; Ikaria, Greece; and Nicoya Peninsula, Costa Rica.

In all these places, people's food choices have one thing in common: They emphasize foods from plant sources. That means sweet potatoes, rice, and vegetables in Okinawa; vegetables, beans, and fruit in Loma Linda; whole-wheat bread, fava beans, and nuts in Sardinia; corn and beans in Costa Rica; bread, olives, greens, and beans in Ikaria.

Fargo, North Dakota, is not a blue zone. Growing up in Fargo, our summers were green, our winters were very white, and you could always smell the sugar beet factory when the wind was in the right direction. My paternal grandfather was a Midwestern rancher. So was my great-grandfather and every generation before that, so far as I could trace. If it walked on four legs, it was likely to end up on the table.

Two legs, too. Ducks and geese flew over the North Dakota wetlands, and every fall my father took his sons out hunting. Eviscerating the smelly carcasses on our cement basement floor, we would not have qualified for *Top Chef.* We had very limited appreciation for vegetables or fruits.

My own meat-laden diet was made worse by my summer job, tending the deep-fryer at McDonald's. By the end of my shift, I probably had more grease soaked into my clothes than Masu ate in an entire month.

Our meal choices didn't help us very much. As I mentioned in chapter 1, all of my grandparents developed severe dementia. The last years of their lives were miserable. So what's the difference between Fargo and Okinawa? Or, for that matter, between Illinois, Iowa, or Kentucky, on the one hand, and Loma Linda or Ikaria, Greece, on the other? Is it just a question of food? Certainly we eat differently. But you have to wonder if some of the credit for the good health people enjoy in the blue zones should go to clean air or genetics.

Researchers at Loma Linda University wondered, too. And they decided to find out. They invited people to join a study and put them into groups of four. Everyone lived in more or less the same area. But each group included one person following a vegetarian diet, one following a vegan diet (no animal products at all), and two people on typical American diets. In all, 272 people were part of the study. And then the researchers just sat back and waited.

What happened next was striking—and it did not say much for California air. Even though everyone lived in the same community, breathed the same air, and had more or less similar genetic risks, those who skipped meat were only *one-third as likely to develop Alzheimer's disease* compared with those who routinely ate meat.[1] Chalk one up for food. While other aspects of a healthy lifestyle are important, as we'll see shortly, it looks like food choices weigh in big.

More Clues from Chicago

In the last chapter, we saw how Chicago researchers had identified copper as a suspect in cognitive decline. The blame, it seems, goes to copper's tendency to accumulate in plaques and produce free radicals that can damage cells. But copper's dangers seemed to depend, oddly enough, on how much fat people were eating. That is, people whose diets included a lot of copper, along with a good dose of *saturated fat* or *partially hydrogenated oils*, were much more likely to lose their mental faculties over time. Those who generally avoided these fats were more likely to stay sharp—regardless of how much copper was in their diets. Copper seemed to be dangerous only when the diet also held a fair amount of saturated fat.

You've seen saturated fat. It is what makes up the white streaks marbling through a chunk of bacon or steak. It is what makes whole milk creamy and cheese waxy. Its name comes from the fact that the fat molecule—if you could look at it under a powerful microscope—is completely covered with hydrogen atoms. That is, it is *saturated* with them. But you don't need to

Alzheimer's Risk from Saturated Fat

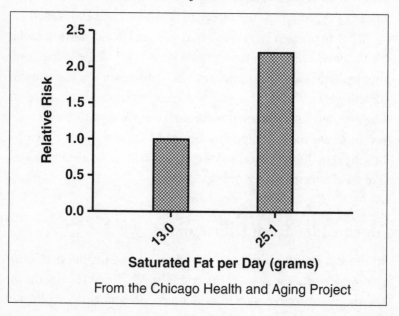

From the Chicago Health and Aging Project

be a chemist to spot saturated fat. At room temperature, it is solid. So lard and cheese are obviously loaded with it, while corn oil and olive oil, which are easily pourable, are not.

In the American diet, the biggest source of saturated fat is from dairy products—cheese, ice cream, butter, and milk. Meats—chicken, sausage, burgers, and roast beef—are a close second.[2]

So copper plus bad fats equals a higher risk of brain problems. However, the Chicago researchers found that saturated fat is apparently harmful *all by itself.* Over a four-year period, people who got around 25 grams of saturated fat each day had at least twice the risk of developing Alzheimer's disease compared with those who got only about half that much.[3] Typical vegetable oils had the opposite effect, reducing the risk of Alzheimer's.

The other "bad" fat is *partially hydrogenated oil,* sometimes called *trans* fat. It is produced by a process called *hydrogenation,* which food manufacturers use to turn liquid oils into solid fats. With a buttery mouthfeel and a long shelf life, these artificial fats are packed into pastries, snack foods, and french fries. Unfortunately, they don't extend *your* shelf life. The Chicago research team found that people consuming the most partially hydrogenated oils had more than double the risk of Alzheimer's compared with people who generally avoid these fats.[3]

Similar findings turned up in New York, where Columbia University researchers tracked 908 elderly New Yorkers. All were free of Alzheimer's disease when the study began. But over the next four years, those who ate the most calories and fat were more than twice as likely to develop Alzheimer's compared with those who ate more modestly.[4] The New York team then brought more volunteers into the study, and much the same pattern held. Those who tended to favor meat and dairy products had a higher risk of developing Alzheimer's disease compared with those who chose what the researchers called a "Mediterranean" pattern of more healthful foods.[5] In both the Chicago and the New York studies, people who had fewer "bad" fats in their diets had less risk, and this was true *even if they had APOE e4 allele.*

A study in Finland came up with much the same result: Saturated fat increased the risk of dementia in people with APOE e4 allele.[6] A Dutch study broke from the pattern, suggesting that diet mattered in the first few years of observation but not after that, for reasons that are not clear.[7] Overall, the jury says that something about the fat in meat and dairy products poses a problem for the brain.

So it looks like these "bad" fats are linked to Alzheimer's disease, and teaming up with copper makes things all the worse.

Compare the Saturated Fat Content

It makes sense to take advantage of foods from plant sources. With few exceptions, foods from plant sources are strikingly low in saturated fat.

HIGH-FAT (IN GRAMS)		LOW-FAT (IN GRAMS)	
Beef, ground (3 oz.)	5.6	Apple (1 medium)	0.1
Cashews (1 oz.)	2.2	Banana (1 medium)	0.1
Cheese, cheddar (1 oz.)	6.0	Beans, pinto (½ cup)	0.2
Cheese, mozzarella (1 oz.)	3.7	Broccoli (1 cup)	0.1
Chicken breast (½ breast, roasted)	2.1	Chickpeas (½ cup)	0.1
		Orange (1 large)	0.0
Egg (1 large)	1.6	Potato (1 medium)	0.1
Milk, whole (1 cup)	4.6	Rice, brown (1 cup)	0.3
Salmon, Atlantic (3 oz.)	2.1		

Bad for the Heart, Bad for the Brain

Saturated fat, trans fats—is some of this sounding familiar? If so, it is because these same "bad" fats assault the heart. Saturated fats and partially hydrogenated oils cause your body to make more cholesterol, which, in turn, encourages plaques to form in the arteries to your heart and to your brain—plaques that gradually pinch off the passage of blood.

If these "bad" fats are a regular part of your diet, your cholesterol level is likely to rise. And studies show that people with high cholesterol levels are more likely to develop Alzheimer's. Compared with a person whose cholesterol level is under 200 milligrams per deciliter, if your cholesterol is around 220, you are not just courting a heart attack. Your Alzheimer's risk is higher, too—about 25 percent higher. And if your cholesterol is in the 250 range or higher, your likelihood of developing Alzheimer's would be about 50 percent higher.[8] These numbers come from a study of 9,844 Kaiser Permanente subscribers in California who had their cholesterols checked when they were in their early forties. *A high cholesterol level in midlife predicted their Alzheimer's risk twenty to thirty years later.*

Understanding Your Cholesterol Test

A high cholesterol level is linked to risk of Alzheimer's disease. Here is how to interpret your own test results:

- Total cholesterol simply means all the various forms of cholesterol added together. According to most authorities, this value should be below 200 milligrams per deciliter (5.2 millimoles per liter). However, for greater safety, some doctors (including me) recommend a limit of 150 milligrams per deciliter (3.9 millimoles per liter) or below.
- Low-density lipoprotein (LDL) cholesterol is also called "bad" cholesterol, because it increases the risk of

(continued)

plaques. It should be below 100 milligrams per deciliter (2.6 millimoles per liter), and some experts suggest an even lower limit of 80 milligrams per deciliter (2.1 millimoles per liter).

- High-density lipoprotein (HDL) cholesterol is referred to as "good" cholesterol, because it carries cholesterol away. It should be above 45 milligrams per deciliter (1.2 millimoles per liter) for men, and above 55 milligrams per deciliter (1.4 millimoles per liter) for women. However, if your total cholesterol is very low (below 150 mg/dL) as the result of a healthful diet, it may be that a low HDL is not a problem. Keep in mind that HDL's function is to carry cholesterol away. So if there is very little cholesterol in your bloodstream, you presumably need less HDL.

- Triglycerides should be below 150 milligrams per deciliter (1.7 millimoles per liter). Triglycerides are particles of fat in the blood and are strongly affected by meals. For this reason, it is best to have your blood test while fasting.

It had once been thought that cholesterol in the bloodstream had nothing to do with cholesterol in the brain;[9] the brain actually makes its own cholesterol. But researchers now believe the situation is not so simple. They are teasing apart the reasons why fat and cholesterol that cause heart problems are linked to brain problems, too.

The Cholesterol Connection

The field of Alzheimer's disease research sometimes feels like a huge jigsaw puzzle where pieces are starting to fit together, even while many gaps remain. Here are some of the pieces researchers are linking together:

- People who eat more saturated fat and partially hydro-genated oils are at higher risk of developing Alzheimer's. Both of these "bad" fats boost cholesterol production in the body, and high cholesterol levels are linked to Alzheimer's risk, too.

- The APOE gene makes a protein that transports choles-terol. It turns out, in fact, to be the *main transporter of cholesterol* within the brain. People who have the e4 ver-sion (allele) of this gene—the version linked to Alzhei-mer's risk—absorb cholesterol more easily from their digestive tracts compared with people who do not have this allele. They tend to have higher cholesterol levels and higher risk of both heart disease and stroke.[10]

- Cholesterol increases the production of beta-amyloid and plays a role in the formation of the beta-amyloid plaques that can lead to Alzheimer's disease.[9]

Suddenly the puzzle is starting to make sense. Toxic fats cause your body to make cholesterol. And cholesterol, carried by the apoE protein, encourages the production of the beta-amyloid that is so hard on your brain cells. Metals aggravate this process, as we saw in the last chapter, with zinc causing the beta-amyloid to clump together and copper and iron making free radicals that destroy our brain cells. And bit by bit, the neuronal connections that recorded your grandchildren's names, what you did yester-day, and what you ate for breakfast start to go haywire.

As biological explanations like this begin to take shape, researchers protest that the jigsaw puzzle is by no means com-plete, and they are right. Even so, the message that emerges is strikingly optimistic. Let's say you have the APOE e4 gene, which busily makes proteins that are eager to escort cholesterol around your body, like so many shopping carts waiting at the meat counter. Presumably you're at risk. Well, what if you were to change your diet? What if you were to bypass the meat counter altogether and favor vegetables, fruits, whole grains, and beans instead? Your body would make less cholesterol, your absorption of metals would diminish, and your risk would fall. Means of protecting ourselves are starting to become clear, even if genes would otherwise be working against us.[3,4,11]

Add It Up

Could it really be that simple? Could toxic fats really push us toward Alzheimer's disease, and could avoiding them make a difference? Well, first, let's understand the numbers. What would it take to get to the amount that turned out to be particularly dangerous in the Chicago study—that is, 25 grams of saturated fat?

It is surprisingly easy. Dairy products, meat, and eggs are loaded with it. So if you had just one egg with bacon for breakfast, a grilled cheese sandwich for lunch, and a moderate serving of meat for dinner, they would add up to 25 grams of "bad" fat.

Or have a glass of milk for breakfast, a serving of salmon for lunch, and half a cheese pizza for dinner. Bingo. You're already at 25 grams of saturated fat.

"Yikes!" I hear you say. "That's the way most people eat!" True enough. The North Dakota breakfasts I grew up on are not looking so good. We had an egg or two every morning, sometimes with bacon or sausage. We never used butter, but we topped our toast with margarine made from partially hydrogenated fat. We poured milk on our cereal and had another glass of milk on the side. My parents led the way, thinking they were providing nutritious meals for themselves and their children.

Sometimes I wonder what would have happened if my grandfather had not raised cattle for a living. It sounds silly to even raise the question, but what if, instead of living on beef, chicken, and milk, our family's staples had been like those in Loma Linda or Okinawa or Sardinia, or any of the other places where people live long, healthy lives? Could the long, slow mental decline that preceded my grandparents' deaths have been prevented?

There is no way of telling for sure. But the good news is that there are plenty of healthful foods that we can take advantage of today. Vegetables, fruits, beans, and grains have essentially no "bad" fats at all. So maybe you'd like Masu's sweet potatoes, rice, and green vegetables, or Ellsworth's baked beans, corn on the cob, and soy yogurt. But how about paging through the recipe section of this book, where you'll find Spiced Pumpkin Bread and Blueberry Buckwheat Pancakes for breakfast, Creamy

---

Diet Versus Drugs

As we've seen, high cholesterol levels are linked to dementia. So you'll want to keep a healthy, low cholesterol level. To do that, I would encourage you to focus on healthful foods and to reserve cholesterol-lowering drugs for when a healthy diet does not bring cholesterol down. So far, drugs do not seem to be able to equal the power of food choices.

Two studies that gave cholesterol-lowering drugs to people over age seventy showed no drop in Alzheimer's risk at all.[12] Now, it could be that the studies were too brief (three and five years, respectively), or perhaps they intervened too late. But the fact is, cholesterol-lowering drugs cannot bring you all the benefits that healthful foods can. Cholesterol medicines don't trim your waistline or lower your blood pressure. They don't have any fiber or healthful vitamins. So while they may be helpful in some cases, they do not take the place of rearranging your refrigerator. In chapter 9, we'll trace out a healthful diet in detail.

Pumpkin Bisque, Easy Colorful Pasta Salad, Sweet Potato Burritos, or White Bean Chili for lunch, followed by Red Lentil or Potato Leek Soup, and Baked Ziti or Risotto Primavera for dinner, with a nice Warm Apple Cherry Compote, Baked Apples, or Chocolate Pudding for dessert? The choices are endless.

Do We Need Meat or Dairy Products?

If the main sources of saturated fat are dairy products and meats, you may be asking, how much meat and dairy products do we actually need?

The answer is, none at all. The healthiest diets exclude animal products completely. I must admit I was slow to come to this realization, which I will blame on my Midwestern upbringing. But studies show that people who choose the veggie burger over the meat variety and top their spaghetti with chunky tomatoes, fresh basil, and asparagus tips instead of meat and cheese get an enormous return on their investment. They are healthier. People who make this change, even late in life, find that excess weight trims away, artery blockages begin to reverse, diabetes improves and sometimes even disappears, blood pressure comes back toward where it ought to be, and their brain cells breathe a huge sigh of relief.

For many people this feels like a tall order. But we have found a way to give you a no-risk test-drive of a 100 percent healthy diet. You'll see it in chapter 9.

"Good" Fats

As we have seen, saturated fat and partially hydrogenated oils are really quite unhelpful. But not all fats are so ill-bred. Some are actually good for you. Here's the reason:

Every cell in your body is surrounded by a cell membrane. This membrane has three layers—two protein layers with a layer of fat sandwiched in between.

If you were to take a close look at this membrane, that fatty middle layer might look unimportant. But it determines a great deal about how the cell works. Imagine that the engine in your car has new, fine motor oil coursing through its moving parts. Everything works great. Now, what if that oil were replaced by thick, black tar? Nothing would work right. Well, the type of fat that is in your cell membranes affects how they work, too. If your cell membranes have "good" fats, they tend to stay healthy.

In 2003, French researchers sampled red blood cells of 246 older people, finding that those whose cell membranes were rich in a certain type of fats, called *omega-3* fats, were more likely to maintain their cognitive functions compared with other people.[13] An earlier study had shown a similar result: A high level of omega-3s in people's blood seemed to protect against cognitive decline and Alzheimer's disease, at least to a degree.[14]

Not every study has shown this benefit,[15] but overall, evidence suggests that having "good" fats in your cell membranes may be helpful. So what are they and how do you get them there?

Let's start by taking a look at a sprig of broccoli. As you look at it, you can see that it doesn't have very much fat, of course. But it actually does have some, surprisingly enough. And there is one particular fat hidden there that your body needs. It is an omega-3 fat called *ALA*, or *alpha-linolenic acid*.

Putting that ALA molecule under a powerful microscope, we see that it is actually a chain of eighteen carbon atoms joined together. If you were to swallow a bit of broccoli, these healthy fat molecules would pass into your bloodstream. Your body would then lengthen the molecular chain from eighteen carbons to twenty, making a new fat called *EPA (eicosapentae-noic acid)*. You would then tack on two more carbons to make the 22-carbon *DHA (docosahexaenoic acid)*. And it is DHA that the brain needs. So it all starts with ALA, the basic "good" fat in food, and you end up with DHA for your brain.

Now, broccoli is just an example. There are traces of ALA in many vegetables, fruits, and beans, and much larger amounts in other foods, especially walnuts, seeds, flax and flax oil, and canola oil. With these foods in your diet, you'll have the raw material for building the fats your brain can use.

But there's a complication here. In order to elongate ALA from eighteen carbons to twenty and eventually to twenty-two carbons—that is, in order to make the fats the brain is looking for—ALA depends on enzymes. Enzymes are the factory workers that take the ALA chain and bolt on the extra carbons to deliver DHA to your brain. And like factory workers everywhere, they can only do so much.

There are certain other fats—called omega-6s—that are just as eager to have extra carbons bolted into place. They tie up the enzymes you need to handle your omega-3s. Omega-6 fats are found in certain cooking oils—safflower oil, sunflower oil, corn oil, cottonseed oil, soybean oil, and grapeseed oil. And there is a whole lot more omega-6 fat in a bottle of any one of these oils than there is omega-3 in broccoli or any other green vegetable. So if you are slathering these oils all over your foods, they slip into your bloodstream and occupy the enzymes that should be handling ALA.[16] And suddenly your brain is wondering what happened to the "good" fats it needs.

Now, you do need a little bit of omega-6. But most people's diets include so much of these oils that they crowd out everything else. Their enzymes are all tied up, and only a fraction of their ALA is ever converted to the longer-chain forms.

So, omega-3s are good, and if you have too much omega-6, it will crowd out your omega-3s. What should you do?

The first step is to have ALA-rich foods in your diet. Have plenty of vegetables, fruits, and beans, and, if you like, top your salad with slivered walnuts or ground flaxseed, for example.

The second step is to greatly limit competing fats. Take a look at the low-fat cooking techniques described in chapter 9 and in the recipe section. You'll be able to sauté onions and garlic without drowning them in grease. And you'll be able to top a salad with lighter, healthier dressings.

You already want to avoid animal fat and partially hydrogenated oils because of the harm they do. Limiting or avoiding cooking oils is a good idea, too.

It's really a question of balance—getting an adequate amount of ALA while limiting the competing oils. The balance your body is looking for is somewhere around 2:1 to 4:1—that is, 2 to 4 grams of omega-6 for every gram of omega-3.[16] That is the ratio that maximizes your body's ability to use the omega-3 to build the longer-chain fats your brain uses. If your menu emphasizes vegetables, fruits, and beans, your foods would give you a pretty good balance of fats naturally. While these healthful foods don't have a great deal of any sort of fat, what they do have is proportionately rich in omega-3s, as opposed to other kinds of fat.

Some people take a third step, which is to make sure they have DHA in their diets. Their rationale is that for most people very little ALA is actually lengthened to EPA and DHA, so they aim to get DHA directly. Their problem, of course, may be that they are getting too much omega-6, and it is tying up their conversion enzymes. So cutting out those competing oils is important. Still, if you do decide to include DHA in your diet, the most healthful source is a DHA supplement, which you will find at any health food store. Vegan brands are preferable. Their DHA is derived from algae rather than from fish, and they contain no animal-derived ingredients.

That said, omega-3 supplements have not yet proved their worth for preventing dementia. In a two-year English study, 867 elderly people were given a capsule that contained two different omega-3s: 200 milligrams of EPA plus 500 milligrams of DHA. It did nothing to forestall memory loss. The participants' reaction time, spatial memory, and processing speed were no better than for people given a placebo.[17] A Dutch study showed the same result.[18] It may be that omega-3 supplements would show more benefit in people who had low omega-3 intake to start with.

Fish oil supplements have also been tested in people who have Alzheimer's disease to see if they can slow the disease process. So far, results are disappointing. An eighteen-month test of fish oil (2 grams of DHA) in Alzheimer's patients showed no benefit.[19]

The take-home message is not to rely on pills. Instead, put omega-3-rich foods on your daily menu.

Skip Fish

Some people take a different approach, choosing foods with more vegetable oils than I have been suggesting and adding fish to their diets. Indeed, compared with beef fat or chicken fat, vegetable oils and fish oils have less saturated fat, and fish has more omega-3 fatty acids. In the Chicago study, people who favored vegetable oils and fish had a reduced risk of dementia compared with people who focused on meatier fare, and several other studies have shown much the same thing.[20,21]

However, a serving of fish is much more like beef than it is like broccoli. As a group, people who eat fish have more weight problems and have a higher risk of diabetes compared with people who skip animal products altogether.[22] And excess body weight and diabetes can both put you at higher risk for Alzheimer's disease. So, if you are already following a healthful plant-based diet, fish is really a step backward.

Part of the problem is that many fish species are fatty. Atlantic salmon, for example, is about 40 percent fat. Chinook salmon is around 50 percent.

"But it's *good* fat," you say. Well, yes, some of it is. But fish fat is always a mixture. About 15 to 30 percent of the fat in fish is omega-3, depending on which species you buy. The other 70 to 85 percent is not "good" fat. It is just a blend of saturated and various unsaturated fats. And every last fat gram packs 9 calories, which is why fatty fish can easily add to your waistline.

Fish also contains cholesterol, just as other animal products do. Some—particularly shellfish like shrimp and lobster—have more cholesterol than red meat. That, plus the methylmercury and other pollutants found in many species (such as tuna), makes fish a less-than-attractive choice. There are other sources of omega-3s that are much more healthful.

It may be that the "benefits" of fish seen in some studies are simply a compensation for the harm of red meat. In other words, fish's anti-inflammatory or anticoagulant tendencies counteract the opposite tendencies of other meats.[23]

Not surprisingly, in the blue zones, fish is not a large part of the diet—not even in Okinawa or Sardinia. The diet staples come from plant sources.

Beyond the Mediterranean

Some people promote a "Mediterranean diet," meaning one that emphasizes vegetables, fruits, beans, and pasta, fish rather than red meat, olive oil instead of butter, and perhaps wine. It's an easy sell. To North Americans, the word "Mediterranean" conjures up sunny images of places they would rather be.

Earlier I mentioned a Columbia University study in which researchers rated the diets of New Yorkers. Those who emphasized vegetables, fruits, legumes, grains, and fish, while having less meat and dairy products, along with mild to moderate alcohol consumption, cut the risk of developing Alzheimer's disease over the next five years by 32 to 40 percent.[5]

The same sort of diet pattern made less difference in a French study.[24] Researchers tracked the health of 1,410 people in Bordeaux, finding that this sort of dietary pattern did not reduce the risk of Alzheimer's disease or other kinds of dementia over the five-year study, although it did seem to slow decline in some cognitive tests.

For most of us, a "Mediterranean diet" pattern is a change in the right direction. It certainly beats the kind of diet I grew up with, and that may be true for you, too. But my assessment is that we can do better. In the same way that people following chicken- or fish-based diets do not do as well as people who avoid meats altogether when it comes to their weight, their diabetes risk, or their heart health, the same is very likely true for brain health as well.

So I would suggest taking the best of the Mediterranean pattern—the vegetables, fruits, beans, and grains—and skipping the fish and oil. We'll talk about alcohol in the next chapter.

Added Bonuses

Avoiding fatty foods and emphasizing healthful plant-based meals brings you a couple of added benefits:

Trimming your waistline. People who eat plant-based

diets are, as a group, much slimmer than people who eat animal products, including fish. Part of the credit goes to the fiber in vegetables, fruits, beans, and whole grains. Fiber satisfies your appetite with essentially no calories. In addition, plant-based diets also tend to slightly increase your metabolism in the after-meal period.[25] As a result, you'll discover that, even though you have not been counting calories or limiting carbohydrates—and even without adding exercise to your routine—a plant-based diet makes it a lot easier to fit into your jeans.[25,26,27]

In turn, that slimmer figure means you'll have less risk of developing diabetes, heart problems, or high blood pressure. And slimmer people also have less risk of Alzheimer's disease.[28]

If you are wondering if your weight is in the healthy range, you can check your body mass index. The BMI is a way of looking at your weight while adjusting for your height. This is important because 140 pounds is a healthy weight if you are five foot seven, but not at all if you are six foot five. You'll find an easy online BMI calculator at www.nhlbisupport.com/bmi/. A healthful BMI is between 18.5 and 25 kg/m².

If you have some weight to lose, let me encourage you *not* to bother with a typical calorie-restricted weight-loss diet. Instead, fill up on vegetables, fruits, whole grains, and legumes, and skip animal products and oily foods, and your weight will adjust itself much more easily. See chapter 9.

Lowering your blood pressure. As you know, diet changes can lower blood pressure. The first step most people try is to reduce salt, which is smart, but usually only modestly effective. A much more powerful step is to avoid fatty foods, especially animal products.[29] This reduces the *viscosity* (thickness) of your blood, so it is less like grease and more like water. That means your blood flows more easily and your heart does not have to work so hard to push blood along. Your blood pressure promptly falls.

And there's more: Fruits and vegetables are rich in potassium, which tends to reduce blood pressure as well. And the weight loss you are enjoying will help bring your pressure down, too.

Together, these steps can have an enormous effect. In chapter 9, I'll show the best way to put all these things together. It's easier than you might guess.

Understanding Your Blood Pressure

Checking your blood pressure, your health-care provider records two numbers (e.g., 120/80). Here is what they mean:

- The first number is your *systolic* blood pressure. It is the wave of pressure that comes with each heartbeat.
- The second number is your *diastolic* blood pressure and represents the relaxation between heartbeats.

A blood pressure below 120/80 is considered normal. A pressure between 120/80 and 140/90 is called prehypertension, and higher values are called hypertension.

So far, we have mostly focused on things to avoid—toxic metals and "bad" fats in particular. But there are certain nutrients that you want to be sure to include in your regular diet—four vitamins that protect your health, including your brain function. In the following chapter, we'll see how they work and where to find them.

CHAPTER 4

Foods That Build Your Vitamin Shield

Avoid toxic metals and "bad" fats—sounds like an easy prescription so far. But we're just getting started. There is a lot more you'll want to do to protect yourself.

Certain critically important vitamins—nutrients that can easily be neglected—play vital roles in protecting your brain. Let's take a look at four of them: vitamin E, folate, vitamin B_6, and vitamin B_{12}.

Vitamin E Protects Against Free Radicals

Vitamin E protects your cells. Specifically, it knocks out free radicals, those angry torpedoes that form, in part, due to copper and iron, as we saw in chapter 2. Vitamin E is an *antioxidant*. It neutralizes free radicals as they arise.

This is important for every part of your body. But it is critical for your brain. Skin cells and muscle cells can be replaced, and red blood cells and white blood cells turn over so quickly, they practically have a sell-by date. But brain cells are forever. Your ability to regenerate new ones is very limited, and there just aren't a lot of shiny new replacement parts ready to stand in for brain cells that have died.

Every brain cell, the axon that extends from it, and the synapses that link it with other cells are fragile. Like an old stone statue in a town square assaulted day after day by air pollutants and acid rain, each brain cell is nicked and pockmarked by the microscopic attacks of free radicals. Vitamin E is a key part of your antioxidant shield.

So, does it work? Does vitamin E actually protect your brain cells? Dutch researchers analyzed the diets of 5,395 people, all of whom were fifty-five or older as the study began. They tracked how much vitamin E they were getting in foods, and they then followed them over the next decade. It turned out that those who got the most vitamin E cut their risk of developing Alzheimer's disease and other forms of dementia by about 25 percent.[1]

Similarly, the Chicago researchers found that in older people followed over a four-year period, Alzheimer's disease developed in 14.3 percent of those who had relatively little vitamin E in their diets, *but in only 5.9 percent of those who got the most vitamin E.*[2] Here is the math: Every 5 milligrams of vitamin E in a person's daily diet reduced the risk of developing Alzheimer's disease by 26 percent.[3]

In the Dutch study, it did not matter if you had the APOE e4 allele—vitamin E was still helpful. But in the Chicago study, it seemed to work only in people who did *not* have the APOE e4 allele, for reasons that are not clear.

Two caveats: First, not all research teams have confirmed the protective effect of vitamin E for the brain. Second, don't rush to the store and buy a bottle of vitamin E. Get it from foods instead. Here is why: Most vitamin E supplements have only one form of the vitamin, called *alpha-tocopherol*. Foods provide it, too, but they also have a second form, called *gamma-tocopherol*, and others as well. These various forms of vitamin E work as a team. There is no need to bother with pills, and some evidence suggests that vitamin E pills are not effective against dementia.[4]

What if you have Alzheimer's already? Will vitamin E help? In 1997, a large research project found that vitamin E did seem to slow the decline of Alzheimer's disease. Called the Alzheimer's Disease Cooperative Study, the project enrolled people with moderately severe symptoms.[5] Their average age was seventy-three, and they had had Alzheimer's disease for about five years. By taking 1000 IU of vitamin E (alpha-tocopherol) twice a day, they were able to delay further decline by nearly two years. "Decline" meant loss of the ability to perform activities of daily living, severe dementia, institutionalization, or death.

Unfortunately, this optimistic finding was not replicated by later studies, and the role of vitamin E in Alzheimer's treatment remains a matter of debate. So, for prevention, vitamin E–rich foods do seem to be effective, but once dementia has begun, its benefits are uncertain.

The recommended dietary allowance for vitamin E for adults is 15 milligrams (22.4 IU) per day. The amount that helped in the Dutch study was around 18.5 milligrams (27.6 IU) per day. The amount that helped in the Chicago study was just 7.6 milligrams (11.4 IU) per day.

Where Do You Find Vitamin E?

You'll find traces of vitamin E in broccoli, spinach, sweet potatoes, mangoes, and avocados. And there is much more in nuts and seeds, especially almonds, walnuts, hazelnuts, pine nuts, pecans, pistachios, sunflower seeds, sesame seeds, and flaxseed.

An ounce of typical nuts or seeds has about 5 milligrams of vitamin E. How much is an ounce? Pour some nuts or seeds into the palm of your hand and stop before they reach your fingers. That is about an ounce. If that's part of your routine, it trims your Alzheimer's risk by about one-quarter, if the Chicago findings hold.

While nuts and seeds are rich in vitamin E, they are also high in fat, which means they pack a lot of calories, not to mention some saturated fat. So I would suggest using them sparingly, focusing on the vitamin E–rich varieties mentioned above rather than peanuts or cashews, which have less vitamin E and more saturated fat.

If you have a tendency to overdo it with nuts and seeds—you tear open a pack and pretty soon you've eaten the whole thing—try this: Use them as an *ingredient,* rather than as a snack food that you might eat all by itself. Sprinkle them on your salad or into a sauce. That way you'll be less tempted to go back for more.

Vitamin E–Rich Foods[6]

GAMMA-TOCOPHEROL		ALPHA-TOCOPHEROL	
Black walnuts	8.1	Sunflower seeds	7.4
Sesame seeds	8.0	Almonds	7.3
Pecans	6.9	Almond butter	6.9
Pistachios	6.4	Hazelnuts	4.3
English walnuts	5.9	Pine nuts	2.6
Flaxseed	5.7	Brazil nuts	1.6

Amounts are listed in milligrams per ounce.

B Vitamins Shield Against Homocysteine

Vitamin E is not the only important nutrient. Three other vitamins are being studied for their role in protecting the brain. Let me tell you what they do.

There is a small, destructive molecule that circulates in your bloodstream, called *homocysteine* (pronounced *ho-mo-SIS-teen*). At high levels, it is linked to risk for heart attacks and strokes. It also affects the brain. Exactly how it does its dirty work is not entirely clear, but some have suggested that, among other things, homocysteine works in combination with copper and cholesterol to damage brain cells.[7]

Where does this nasty actor come from? Well, you don't inhale it, you don't drink it, and it does not come from food. It is actually created *within your body*. As your cells build protein, homocysteine is a temporary by-product made along the way.

That's where vitamins come in. They help you get rid of it. Specifically, three B vitamins—vitamin B_6, vitamin B_{12}, and folate—work as a team to eliminate homocysteine. If you are low in any one of them, it will tend to build up in your bloodstream.

In the Netherlands, researchers conducted a study to see what folate supplements could do to boost memory and cognition overall.[8] They invited a group of volunteers to participate. They were healthy, between fifty and seventy years of age, and free of any major memory problems, but they all had high homocysteine levels on blood tests. Everyone was asked to complete some basic cognitive tests. For example, they were given a list of fifteen words and asked to recall as many as they could twenty minutes later. They were asked to name as many animals as they could think of in one minute. The researchers measured their reaction times.

Then, half the volunteers were given folate supplements of 800 micrograms per day. The other half were given a placebo—a dummy pill that had no folate in it at all. Every year for the next three years, they were tested again.

The placebo group ended up getting no benefits, needless to say. But for the folate group, homocysteine levels promptly fell, from around 13 micromoles per liter to around 10. Their memories improved, and they were thinking measurably more quickly compared to participants who did not get folate.

Note that the people in the Netherlands were within the range of what we would consider normal mental functioning. Even so, folate made a noticeable difference.

Researchers at Oxford University went a step further, testing folate, vitamin B_6, and vitamin B_{12} in older people who were having memory problems that were sufficient for a diagnosis of mild cognitive impairment.[9] As you will recall, that means they had significant forgetfulness but were otherwise fine for the moment. The researchers gave everyone a set of cognitive tests. Then, over the next two years, the participants started a

---

Folate and Hearing

The Dutch researchers who found that folate could help memory and cognition also looked to see what it might do for hearing.[10] After all, gradual hearing loss is something many people experience in older age. In the three-year study, the placebo group had the usual gradual drop-off in hearing, which was not surprising. But the people taking folate had considerably less hearing loss at the frequencies associated with speech. There was not any benefit at high frequencies.

This does not mean that folate *improves* damaged hearing. But it does mean that it may help you keep the hearing you have.

daily regimen that consisted of 800 micrograms of folate, 500 micrograms of vitamin B_{12}, and 20 milligrams of vitamin B_6, all of which are well above the recommended dietary allowances for these vitamins and more than one would typically get from foods.

The effects were remarkable. High homocysteine levels fell sharply, and many people found their memory improving significantly. Accuracy on testing was improved by as much as 70 percent. And brain scans showed that the B vitamins also helped protect against brain shrinkage over time.

Can these three vitamins prevent Alzheimer's disease? That is not so clear. But studies of Alzheimer's patients have shown that many have had excess homocysteine levels, suggesting that it is critically important to get the vitamins that eliminate it.[11,12]

Once people have been diagnosed with Alzheimer's disease, vitamin supplementation has been disappointing. In a recent US study involving 409 people with mild to moderate Alzheimer's disease, B_6, B_{12}, and folate supplements showed no benefits for the group as a whole. However, focusing on those whose symptoms were mildest, the vitamins did seem to slow cognitive decline over an eighteen-month period compared with people given a placebo.[13]

Before You Race Out to Buy Supplements

Overall, these studies suggest that folate, B_6, and B_{12} help lower homocysteine, and that helps protect your memory. But before you start loading your shopping cart with supplement bottles, let me share some important caveats:

First, it is likely that benefits of vitamin supplementation will show up in people whose homocysteine levels have been too high as opposed to people with normal homocysteine levels.[8,14]

It is easy for a doctor to check your homocysteine level. A value over 15 micromoles per liter is too high, and some clinicians would call for a more conservative cutoff of 13. If you are in the normal range, it is not necessary to get heroic amounts of these vitamins in your diet. Rather, you just want to make sure you're not missing them.

Second, in the United States, many foods are supplemented with folate. If you are already getting plenty, more is not necessarily better. In fact, overdoing it with folate supplements may well be harmful. In the Chicago study, getting extra folate was not helpful and, if anything, increased the risk of Alzheimer's disease over time.[15] Similarly, in a large Norwegian study, B vitamins were used in people who had recently had heart attacks to see if they could prevent recurrences. However, the study participants did not necessarily have high homocysteine levels, and B vitamins ended up doing more harm than good, boosting the risk of future heart problems by about 20 percent.[16]

So what's the safe and smart way to get the vitamins you need? Let's take them one by one:

Best sources of folate: Folate is in foods with *foliage*—that is, broccoli, spinach, asparagus, and other green leafy vegetables. You'll also find it in beans, peas, citrus fruits, and cantaloupe. It is in all common multivitamin supplements, and, by law, many grain products in the United States are now fortified with it: bread, breakfast cereals, flour, pasta, and rice. The recommended dietary allowance for adults is 400 micrograms per day.

Folate is fragile. With processing and prolonged storage, the folate in foods gradually disappears. So fresh produce—and produce that is frozen quickly after harvest—is a good choice.

Best sources of vitamin B$_6$: Whole grains, green vegetables, beans, sweet potatoes, bananas, and nuts are rich in B$_6$.

If these foods are part of your routine, you will easily meet the recommended dietary allowance. The recommended dietary allowance for B_6 for adults up to age fifty is 1.3 milligrams per day. If you are over fifty, the RDA is 1.5 milligrams for women and 1.7 milligrams for men.

As you have noticed, greens and beans are good sources of both folate and B_6, so you will want to be sure to keep them on your shopping list and on the menu.

Best sources of vitamin B_{12}: B_{12} is in fortified products, such as breakfast cereals or fortified soy milk, in all common multivitamins, and in B_{12} supplements. It is also found in animal-derived products, but the absorption from supplements and fortified foods is much better.

The recommended dietary allowance for adults is 2.4 micrograms. Most supplements have more than that, sometimes much more, and it is not toxic at higher intakes. The US government recommends that everyone over the age of fifty take a B_{12} supplement or choose B_{12}-fortified foods. My advice is that you not wait until you are fifty. A B_{12} supplement is essential for people who avoid animal products and an excellent idea for everyone else, too.

In 2009, a team of researchers in Singapore reported that people who had more vitamin B_{12} circulating in their blood had better memory function and better ability to pay attention. But they also found that B_{12} was especially critical in people with the APOE e4 gene.[17] Those with the APOE e4 gene who were low in B_{12} did badly on memory tests. But people with the APOE e4 gene who had higher B_{12} levels performed much better.

So why would anyone ever run low in B_{12}? Two reasons:

First, poor absorption. The vitamin B_{12} found in animal-derived products is bound to protein, and many people, particularly older people, do not produce enough stomach acid to free B_{12} from the foods that contain it. Acid-blocking medicines, metformin (a common diabetes drug), and stomach disorders can reduce your absorption of vitamin B_{12} even further.

Second, diet. If you are skipping animal products (which is a very good idea), it is essential to have supplemental B_{12}, because foods from plants are devoid of B_{12}, except when they are fortified with it. That said, it is easy to find in B_{12} supplements and fortified foods.

Bottom line: Be sure to have folate, B_6, and B_{12} in your routine. I'd suggest emphasizing green leafy vegetables, beans, and whole grains, and also taking a supplement for B_{12}. They will work together to eliminate homocysteine, protecting your heart and brain.

The Magic of Fruits and Vegetables

By now, you have no doubt noticed that researchers are keen on fruits and vegetables. These healthful foods are loaded with important vitamins and other nutrients, as well as being strikingly low in "bad" fats.

Fortunately, many people share the researchers' enthusiasm. Participants in the Chicago study who got three or four vegetable servings per day slowed their rate of cognitive decline by 40 percent compared with those who got only about one serving of vegetables per day.[18] Fruits and vegetables also help prevent stroke.[19,20]

Are some fruits or vegetables better than others? Are you better off having an apple or a serving of spinach? A team of Dutch researchers tackled that question by analyzing the diets of 20,069 healthy people and then following them for the next ten years to see which foods had the most health power. It turned out that orange fruits and vegetables had the most heart-

protecting power. People who ate the most carrots, sweet potatoes, cantaloupe, butternut squash, and their botanical cousins
cut their risk of heart problems by 26 percent, presumably due
to the beta-carotene and other nutrients in these foods.[21]

When it came to preventing stroke, the real standouts were
apples and pears.[22] People who averaged the equivalent of an
apple a day were able to cut their stroke risk by 50 percent or
more.

But don't focus just on carrots and apples. Go for the variety nature provides. As you walk into the produce section of a
grocery store, you can't help but notice the bright colors. The
orange beta-carotene in carrots and sweet potatoes is a powerful antioxidant. The red color in tomatoes is *lycopene*—a cousin
of beta-carotene and a powerful antioxidant in its own right.
There are many others.

So by all means do have carrots and apples, and have many
other fruits and vegetables, as well. It's the generous variety of
vegetables and fruits in your daily routine that does the trick.

Fruit Juices and Extracts

While you're in the produce section, pick up some berries. Yes,
cranberry juice really does help prevent urinary infections, and
blueberries may do the same. Many berry varieties contain antioxidants and other compounds that counter inflammation, and
researchers have put them to the test for their effects on the
brain. In a small study, researchers at the University of Cincinnati
gave Concord grape juice to people with mild cognitive impairment and found that it improved their learning ability and modestly boosted short-term memory. The amount was roughly one
pint of juice each day for twelve weeks.[23] It was not necessary to
drink it all at once; it could be divided into smaller servings.

The Cincinnati team also found benefit from blueberry juice.[24] These studies were small, and it is not certain that other research studies will confirm their findings. Even so, berries and grapes are healthful foods that are rich in antioxidants with no harmful side effects.

So, Is Wine in the Fruit Group?

In southwestern France, the river Garonne is flanked with vineyards that produce close to a *billion* bottles of wine every year. It is the wine capital of the world. In 2004, researchers in Bordeaux found that people who had a glass or two of wine each day were half as likely to develop Alzheimer's disease compared with teetotalers.[25] They were also less likely to develop other kinds of dementia, such as that caused by strokes.

Now, one might have been tempted to chalk up the findings to a local product promotion. But studies in the Netherlands and New York showed the same benefit—modest drinking cuts the risk of Alzheimer's by about half.

Red wine is unusual in that the prolonged contact of the grape skins with the juice during fermentation lends a deep red color to the wine and also infuses it with bioactive compounds. One, called *resveratrol*, is being studied for antiaging and heart-protective effects. But when it comes to Alzheimer's disease, *any* sort of alcohol seemed to produce the same benefit. It does not have to be wine. A modest intake of alcohol is known to help protect the heart, and it looks like it has the same effect on the brain.

But before you toast to health and longevity, let me offer a couple of caveats.

First, alcohol is not essential for health. People in Loma Linda generally avoid alcohol, because it is discouraged by the

Seventh-day Adventist Church. And yet they do extraordinarily well. In fact, it may be that alcohol's role in other populations is simply to counteract some negative effect of a less-than-healthy diet. If you're eating well, it's not clear that alcohol adds anything.

Second, alcohol has risks. If you're drinking more than about one to two drinks per day, you are at risk for liver disease, accidents, social problems, and several forms of cancer. In fact, the French government has been trying very hard for years to rein in the epidemics of cirrhosis and automobile fatalities that are caused by alcohol.

Even one drink per day—if it is every day—increases a woman's risk of breast cancer. The explanation might be that alcohol interferes with folate. It turns out that the B vitamin that is important for eliminating homocysteine is also part of the body's anticancer defenses, and alcohol disrupts its action.

Alcohol also increases iron absorption. While that may sound helpful, alcohol can contribute to iron overload, especially if you have more than two drinks per day.[26]

So, as you can see, alcohol's effects are complicated and mixed. If you drink alcohol, the best advice is to have it modestly and intermittently as opposed to every day. And be sure to include plenty of greens and beans in your regular diet to give you the folate you need.

Is Coffee in the Bean Group?

In 2010, a team of Finnish researchers found an unusual ally in the battle against Alzheimer's disease: coffee. Over a twenty-one-year period, they tracked the coffee habits of a group of 1,409 people. Some loved it and others avoided it, like everywhere else. But the coffee lovers came out on top, with 64 percent less risk of developing Alzheimer's disease. Even among people carrying the APOE e4 allele, the effect of coffee was clear: a nearly two-thirds drop in their risk![27]

That's great news for coffee drinkers, needless to say. But there are two hitches. First, not every study agrees, although several previous studies did favor coffee, too. Second, only people who drank a lot of coffee—three to five cups a day—showed any benefit, and it looks like decaf doesn't cut it.

Exactly why coffee should help prevent Alzheimer's is still very much up in the air. Caffeine is a stimulant, of course. Coffee also contains antioxidants and dozens of other chemical compounds ready to take credit.

So far, evidence for any benefit from other caffeine-containing beverages, such as tea, is much weaker. As we saw above, tea contains traces of aluminum, which remains a consideration.

There is, of course, a downside to caffeine. It can disrupt your sleep, which, in turn, can harm your memory. It can also make you irritable and even aggravate problems with heart rhythm. Caffeine's effects vary from person to person, so I suggest that you see how it affects you.

A Menu for a Strong Memory

As we have seen in the past three chapters, protecting your memory starts with three improvements to the menu:

1. Shield Yourself from Toxic Metals

You'll want to limit exposure to copper, iron, and zinc, and there is no reason to expose yourself to aluminum at all. With a few judicious choices when it comes to food products, cookware, multiple vitamins, antacids, and so on, you will have enormous control over these potential toxins.

2. Give Your Brain an Oil Change

We need to stop the attack of toxic fats and give your brain the traces of healthy fats it needs. That means shifting from a diet based on meat, cheese, and other animal products to a plant-based menu and avoiding the partially hydrogenated oils that turn up in snack foods and fried foods. As you choose your foods, it pays to be generous with vegetables—especially the green leafy varieties—as well as fruits, legumes, and whole grains.

Skip the cooking oils. In chapter 9, I'll show you simple techniques that allow you to go beyond oil-based cooking.

3. Build Your Vitamin Shield

Four vitamins are key here: vitamin E and three B vitamins.

- For vitamin E, have some broccoli, spinach, sweet potatoes, mangoes, or avocados. Or, for a bigger dose, try almonds, walnuts, hazelnuts, pine nuts, pecans, pistachios, sunflower seeds, sesame seeds, or flaxseed. A small handful of nuts or seeds (about 1 ounce) sprinkled on your salad is a good idea.

Next, be sure to get your B vitamins:

- Folate is in green leafy vegetables, as well as beans, peas, citrus fruits, cantaloupe, and fortified grain products.
- Vitamin B_6 is in beans, green vegetables, bananas, nuts, sweet potatoes, and many vegetables, and also in whole grains.
- Vitamin B_{12} should come in the form of a supplement or fortified foods.

The good news is that the diet changes that may protect your brain are remarkably similar to those that are good for your heart. And they help trim away unwanted weight in the bargain. If you happen to have high blood pressure, diabetes, or cholesterol problems, a healthful plant-based diet can help enormously. A simple set of menu changes accomplishes all of this at one time. In chapter 9, we'll pull it all together in an easy-to-follow menu plan, followed by many recipes to get you started.

In Case You Thought It Was Too Late

By now, you might be thinking, "A healthier diet probably would have been really good for me. But it's too late now. The damage has been done." Let me tell you about someone who decided *not* to say that.

Benjamin Spock, MD, was the world's best-known pediatrician. His book *Baby and Child Care* revolutionized how parents thought about raising children and remains one of the best-selling books of all time.

He was a tall man, strong and athletic, and won an Olympic gold medal with the Yale rowing crew at the 1924 games. Graduating at the top of his class at Columbia University's College of Physicians and Surgeons, he specialized in pediatrics and went on to study psychoanalysis for six years.

But later in life, his health began to fail. In 1991, he began to suffer from chronic lung problems—a recurrent pneumonia that he could not shake. He had had a prior exposure to tuberculosis, and accumulating fluid around his heart and lungs left him vulnerable to chronic infections that antibiotics could not clear. Around the same time, a case of serious food poisoning left him with chronic neuropathy, weakening his legs. His energy was shot.

His doctors at Boston's New England Medical Center had no effective treatment for his worsening health problems. Essentially, they gave up. After all, Ben was in his eighties, and he should not expect miracles. Stay home, buy a wheelchair, and install an elevator, his doctors told him. You've lived a good life.

That didn't sit well with Ben. It was not the implication that he ought to just wait to die that troubled him; it was when he saw the price of installing an elevator that he got steamed!

With the encouragement of his wife, Mary, he decided to try a different approach, which involved taking a long look at his diet and making some major changes. He consulted with a knowledgeable nutritionist, who felt that it was not too late to try something new. Out with the meaty, cheesy junk food, and in with the vegetables and whole grains. Mary kept him on track, preparing soup, rice, stir-fried vegetables, and many other dishes.

Within days, he started to sleep better. By the three-week mark, his strength and energy were back. By six weeks, he had lost fifty pounds of fluid and felt like a new man.

It was not always smooth sailing, however. At a restaurant one night, he was tempted by the menu and decided to "treat" himself to steak. Almost instantly, he felt sick again. His energy was gone and his sleep was disrupted—and that proved to him that it really was the healthy food that had made the difference. He got back on track and felt good again.

Shortly thereafter, he went back to the New England Medical Center—not for a medical appointment this time, but as an invited speaker—and he saw the physicians who had consulted with him before. They were stunned to see his dramatic improvement.

After these life-changing experiences, Dr. Spock began to advocate for a healthful diet. He rewrote *Baby and Child Care* to include information about the value of plant-based diets and getting away from meat and milk—foods he had once thought were essential for children. He worked with my organization, the Physicians Committee for Responsible Medicine, as we pushed the federal government to change its dietary policies.

Speaking with Dr. Spock in his nineties was like talking to a young man embarking on a new adventure. He had a vast knowledge, generous disposition, and a sense of purpose that never left him. Mentally clear every day of his life, he died just shy of his ninety-fifth birthday.

Step II

STRENGTHEN YOUR BRAIN

In the same way that exercise can build muscular strength and endurance, you can do the same thing for your brain.

Cognitive exercises can strengthen synapses—the bridges that connect one brain cell to the next. The more solid these connections, the better off you'll be.

Physical exercises increase blood flow to your brain and actually have been shown to reverse age-related brain shrinkage. Even if you haven't thought about physical activity in some time, there is a new twist on exercise that makes it surprisingly easy. We'll start slowly, take it gently, and you'll be in control every step of the way.

As you'll see, the food choices you learned about in Step One work hand in hand with the simple exercises you'll learn about now in Step Two. The benefits for brain function have been proven in controlled tests and scans of brain structure.

CHAPTER 5

Mental Exercises That Build Your Cognitive Reserve

In a huge, airy loft on Kearny Street in downtown San Francisco, a young man is hunched over a computer screen. Near the top of the screen, a raindrop appears and slowly descends toward the bottom. Written on the raindrop is a bit of arithmetic. It says 9 + 2. The young man quickly punches the number 11 onto the keyboard, and the raindrop explodes into pieces.

Another drop appears. This one says 6 x 1. He punches 6 into the keyboard, and that raindrop explodes as well. Then another says 34 + 10, and he punches in 44. Away it goes. The drops start coming faster and faster, some on the left and others on the right. Intently focused, he reacts as quickly as he can, scoring points for each correct answer.

Next to him, a young woman is looking at a computer screen, too. But hers shows animated human figures. They appear to be customers at a food counter, and they are looking at her expectantly. She has to remember their names and what they've ordered. When she gets them right, she gets a tip.

Across the room, another woman is seated at a computer that is displaying three letters. It says "CAP." She types "cape," "caps," "captain," "capsize," and "capture," and then pauses to think of more words with the same three-letter beginning. The more words she comes up with within the allotted time, the more points she earns.

These people are not playing video games. They are part of a team of computer experts and graphic designers. They are working on a training program that builds what scientists call *cognitive reserve*. It is a new concept in neurology, and one that may help us hold on to memories for much longer.

Building Your Brain Circuits

Not long ago, researchers made a striking observation: Using special neuroimaging techniques, they looked into the brains of living people and found that many of them had quite a lot of amyloid plaques—the microscopic abnormalities that lead to Alzheimer's disease. But despite their ominous-looking scans, some of these people showed no signs of any cognitive problems at all, so far as anyone could tell. They could balance their checkbooks and pay their bills, and they did not stumble over their grandchildren's names.[1] Despite changes in their brains, they somehow managed to keep their memories more or less intact.

How did they do it? The reason, scientists speculate, is intellectual stimulation. By giving their brains constant input over the years, they had built up so many connections between brain cells that they could compensate for losses later on. This is cognitive reserve.

Think of it like a highway. You've got your regular route that leads to your destination. But what if the road ahead is blocked? It helps if you know of a detour or maybe have a choice of several alternate ways you could take. Something similar happens in your brain. If you lose some brain cells or synapses, it is great if other cells or cell connections can get your messages through. The theory is that the more connections you have between cells, the more options you can use in case any start malfunctioning.

So how do you build cognitive reserve? The most obvious way is in your years at school. Yes, all that time plowing through books, working at the blackboard, writing essays, solving math problems, and studying for tests really does strengthen connections in your brain. Indeed, a large study of older adults living in Memphis, Tennessee, and Pittsburgh, Pennsylvania, showed that people with higher levels of education were more likely to retain their mental clarity into old age, compared with people with little education or low literacy levels.[2] Other studies had shown much the same thing. Well-educated people have more "alternate routes" ready in case they need them.

Here's what this might look like from your brain's point of view: You're out with some friends, and someone asks who starred in *Gone with the Wind*. "I can see her face," you say. "But what the heck is her name? It's on the tip of my tongue. She was one of the most famous actresses. . . ."

If you had seen the movie, you may or may not remember the star's name. But what if your brain happened to have laid down a few extra connections? Your brain suddenly starts coughing up all the bits of information it has stored, one linked to the next. The movie was set in the Old South . . . the plantation was called Tara . . . the Civil War was brewing . . . it came out just before World War II . . . what's-her-name was in love with Ashley . . . Ashley went off to war . . . she ended up destitute and married Rhett Butler . . . frankly, my dear, I don't give a damn . . .

that was Clark Gable...Clark Gable and Vivien Leigh....Oh yeah! That's her!

It's not pretty, but out of that salad of ideas comes the name you're looking for. The more connections you've made, the more likely you are to remember things.

Education is good. But you do not need a PhD in nuclear physics. Whatever education you had or didn't have in the past, the activities you do *now* can make a difference. In the Chicago study, even simple mental activities, if done often enough, helped prevent Alzheimer's. That could mean reading a newspaper, a book, or a magazine; working a crossword puzzle; playing cards or checkers; going to a museum; and even watching television or listening to the radio—as long as it's something else that gets your neurons firing. Over a four-year period in Chicago, people who were engaged in these activities the most cut their risk of developing Alzheimer's by about two-thirds compared to people who got very little mental stimulation.[3]

That was encouraging. So a team of researchers developed a specific set of brain-training exercises to see if they could prevent mental decline in older folks. The project was called the ACTIVE study, short for Advanced Cognitive Training for Independent and Vital Elderly.[4] The researchers, from Alabama, Michigan, Massachusetts, Indiana, Maryland, and Pennsylvania, invited a group of 2,832 older adults to participate.

Each participant received up to ten training sessions in memory, reasoning, or processing speed. Some had to remember word lists or do other memory tests. Others were asked to identify patterns in series of letters or words (such as: a...c...e... g...i...). And still others were asked to remember the locations of items that flashed briefly on a computer screen and then vanished. The researchers also gave the participants booster training later on.

Five years later, the participants were tested. And indeed, they were noticeably sharper. How much sharper? They were able to essentially counteract seven to fourteen years of aging.

However, their mental strength was most evident for the *specific areas in which they had been trained*. If they were trained in memory, they did well on memory tests. If they were trained in reasoning, they did well on problem-solving tests. If they had worked on reaction time, they did well on speed tests. These are all separate mental functions, so it makes sense to have a variety of activities that exercise all your mental functions.

In the loft in San Francisco, that is exactly what the computer team is building. This is Lumos Labs, a company that has worked with scientists at major universities to develop a sophisticated set of web-based teaching tools that strengthen memory, attention, reaction speed, and problem solving.

Researchers at the University of New South Wales in Australia used these exercises to see if they could boost mental functioning for people with mild cognitive impairment. In thirty training sessions over twelve weeks, the participants worked on focusing their attention and improving their memory and reaction time. And, indeed, week by week, their performance on each task improved noticeably.

Many different research teams have been testing similar programs to boost flagging cognitive skills. Some researchers do their training in groups, others one-on-one. In 2010, researchers in Quebec sized up the results.[5] And indeed, cognitive training seems to help. It boosts memory, as well as mood and overall quality of life.

To get a feel for this kind of training, take a look at the Lumosity website (Lumosity.com) or the Vivity Labs site (Fit Brains.com). There are dozens of programs. Each one starts out very easy and gradually builds to whatever degree of complexity you could want. If you like, you can subscribe to these services and do the exercises on a regular basis. You can almost feel your brain creating new synapses as you go.

The Bilingual Advantage

One type of mental stimulation is particularly intriguing: being able to speak more than one language. Researchers in Toronto found that bilingual adults are able to buy themselves a little time when it comes to dementia. It is not that they are exempt from brain disorders. But whatever memory problems they may have show up about five years later compared with people who speak only one language.[6]

Similar findings turned up in other studies and with various languages.[7,8] And when it comes to delaying Alzheimer's disease, speaking three languages is better than two, and speaking four beats speaking three.[7]

This makes sense. After all, one of the most common complaints of people with memory problems is the inability to come up with words or names. They'll pause, embarrassed, waiting for the words to emerge from wherever they have been hiding. But if you've been working all your life, not with just one set of words for everything but with two or three, you can imagine the circuitry that you've built up over the years.

Unfortunately, your long-forgotten high school French classes are not much use. What counts is actually *using* languages. That is what keeps the brain limber. We don't yet know if acquiring a second language late in life is as good as growing up bilingual, but I'd suggest hedging your bets and ordering up some language discs or calling your travel agent and booking an immersion week abroad.

Of course, acquiring a new language and learning about

other cultures is mind-expanding in every way, and nowadays it is easier than ever. You can tune in to television broadcasts in many languages. You can learn French by phone (www.French ByPhone.com), study Spanish or Chinese through song lyrics (www.Yabla.com), and learn Vietnamese basics through free online classes (EverydayViet.com). And you'll find every imaginable language book and disc at bookstores and on the web.

Personally, I am hoping to get some credit for growing up in North Dakota, where everyone is essentially bilingual, thanks to the large number of people of Norwegian ancestry. Being bilingual in Fargo was actually quite easy, since we used the same words for nearly everything. "My, it's cold!" would be translated as "Uff da!" If it were hot, we would wipe our brows and sigh "Uff da!" And if English speakers would observe, "Good heavens, that's a pricey meal!" we would turn to each other with a very knowing "Uff da!" As you can see, we were even able to *think* bilingually from earliest age.

Our vocabulary did wander slightly further. We had *lefse,* a flat potato bread smeared with butter and sugar; *krumkake,* which means "bent cake"; and, if you had the courage, *lutefisk,* a cod gelatinized by a lengthy treatment with lye, a process invented centuries ago by someone whose descendants are no doubt still in hiding. Eating these foods would make you feel quite intercultural. Their effect on your brain, however, might undo whatever benefit you might get from bilingualism.

A Simple Memory Aid: Linking

It's 4 a.m. and you were just jerked out of dreamland by the realization that it's tax day and you have not yet mailed in your return. "Uh-oh," you're thinking. "Good thing I remembered." But as you lie there, it hits you that you also need to pick up your shirts at the cleaners and get the car inspected before you go on vacation. It's a lot to remember in the middle of the night. You hate to turn on the light and root around for a pen, knowing you'll never be able to go back to sleep, but you don't dare forget.

This sort of thing happens to us all the time. We need to remember something important, but it's not a handy time to deal with it or to write it down. Let me show you a simple trick.

We'll take a lesson from Ben Pridmore. Ben lives in Derby, in northern England, and he is a memory champion. Ben can memorize a pack of fifty-two cards in less than thirty seconds. You can shuffle them any way you want, hand him the pack, and, after glancing through it, he will look you in the eye and tell you, "two of clubs, queen of hearts, ten of diamonds," and so on through the whole pack, every card in perfect order.

Shuffle again, and Ben will do it all for you once more. How does he do this? Ben is quite happy to tell you: He links mental images.

Here's a simple example: Start with a visual image. It could be any object that you can easily remember and that you associate with things that need doing. For me, that's my little black schedule book where I keep my weekly agenda, phone numbers, and so on. If I happen to wake up in the middle of the night and need to remember something, I start with a mental image of my schedule book. Then I make an image of whatever I need to remember and attach it to the image of the book. So "tax" could become an image of thumbtacks, and I might imagine them sticking into the black schedule book. To make them especially memorable, I'll imagine bright pink or glowing orange tacks. Waking up later, I'll say to myself, "What was I supposed to remember?" I'll go to my mental image of the schedule book and see the odd image of pink thumbtacks and soon realize that I am supposed to send in my tax return.

Let's go a step further. You can link images in a chain. So if I have to remember to mail in a tax return, pick up my shirts, and have the car inspected, the mental image will start with my schedule book, which is the anchor I use every time. Then I'll mentally stick tacks into it and make them a bright memorable color. Then one of the tacks will be nailing a shirt to my schedule book. I'll make the shirts a very memorable color, too. So glowing orange tacks will be sticking a gaudy green shirt to my schedule book. Then I'll add a car that will be driving out of one of the sleeves in a big cloud of smoke. The images should not be logical or mundane. The more nonsensical and graphic they are, the more memorable they will be.

All of this takes just a few seconds. And if the images are striking enough and connected to each other, you can doze off to sleep and easily remember everything later on. Try it, you'll see.

So what does Ben Pridmore do? His system for creating images is considerably more complicated than my middle-of-the-night tacks and shirts, and it requires a bit of practice. But it's basically the same idea. Instead of using a black schedule book as a starting mental image, he mentally "places" images in his grandmother's house, with one image leading to the next.

The images themselves come from a sort of language he devised, in which the playing cards' suits and values spell out the names of simple objects. And it is these objects that he mentally "places" at the various points in his mental journey through his grandmother's house. If you'd like to learn Ben's "language," you'll find it on the Internet, at memoryconsulting.com/prid more.htm.

This is obviously much more challenging than remembering a few simple errands. But it works. Using similar methods, Ben has memorized the value of *pi*—that mathematical value that

our geometry teachers felt was so important—out to 50,000 dig-
its. He starts out with 3.14159…and doesn't quit for hours.

There is certainly no need for you to go to such lengths.
But I raise this to make a point. Your memory is not a jumble,
like a laundry basket or a drawer of socks. When your brain
stores things away, it *connects* them in a chain. And remembering them *depends on connections*, too. Ben could not remember
a single card without connecting it to something—some kind of
mental image. By linking each new memory to an existing one,
the process can go on, more or less indefinitely.

Here's why this matters. Have you ever been introduced to
someone and you soon realize that you had forgotten his or her
name as soon as you heard it? That's because you tossed the
name into your mental laundry basket, hoping you could find
it later. But your brain does not work that way. Any new name,
fact, date, phone number, or anything else that is not linked
to a preexisting spot in your brain will immediately just slide
right out.

So as you say, "Pleased to meet you, Sidney," you'll need
to connect your new friend's name to something. Picture him
at the Sydney opera house with its famous scalloped roofs, or
imagine him skidding on his knees—anything that brings SID-
NEY to mind. Make it graphic (you don't have to tell him what
you came up with).

Professor Jackson can have a ball and jacks on his head (in
your mind). Again, the more graphic it is, the better. Later on,
chances are you'll remember their names.

Memory experts connect people's names to some aspect of
their faces—their noses, their eyes, their ears, or whatever. For
example, meeting a man named Robert, you notice that he has
a rather long nose. It's nothing out of the ordinary, but it is the
first thing you saw. That's where you'll hook your mental pic-

ture. So, to suggest "Robert," you could make an image of a robber and link it to his nose.

The key is to make the images really striking. That means colorful, illogical, sexy, aggressive, or anything else that brings emotion into the mix. So picture a long chain of robbers in striped prison suits running in one nostril and out the other. Bring it into sharp focus. Picture the robbers leaving muddy footprints on his face as they run. Pump up the imagery. When you next see Robert, this image will pop into your mind and will suggest the name.

Mundane images do not work; they trigger the brain's delete button. If that surprises you, think about what your brain conjures up in dreams. Did you ever dream that you did your grocery shopping? Or that you went to work and had a good couple of meetings? Or that you had a successful golf game, that you had a nice dinner with friends, or that you read the newspaper? The answer likely is no, because your brain's scriptwriter thought that all these ideas were too dull and dumped them in favor of images that are poignant, funny, sexy, or loaded with emotion in some other way. Positive emotions are best, because you will want to retain them. If you want to remember something, color it in some way that makes it striking.

There are many books on these techniques. One of the best is Benjamin Levy's *Remember Every Name Every Time* (Fireside, New York, 2002). You'll also find a concise guide to many memory methods in Tony Buzan's *Use Your Perfect Memory* (Plume, New York, 1991).

A Touch of Humility

As exciting as the concept of cognitive reserve is and as useful as memory exercises can be, they do not take the place of physically taking care of yourself. That means eating health-fully and exercising to the extent you can. If you are not eating well—if you are dosing your brain with "bad" fats and toxic metals—the cognitive reserve you have built can be easily and quickly destroyed. Ditto if you are sitting idly instead of getting your heart pumping on a regular basis.

My father went to medical school, finished an internal medicine residency, plowed through every issue of *JAMA* and the *New England Journal of Medicine*, and read the local newspaper every night. Yes, it was the Fargo paper, but it still counts. He built up an enormous cognitive reserve.

But he also grew up on a cattle ranch and never left the taste for beef behind him, except for a few years when my mother managed to convince them both to eat better, before a move into a retirement home made them abandon healthy eating in favor of whatever was on the enjoy-your-golden-years menu for the day. His diet overdosed him with saturated fat and cholesterol, along with iron, copper, and zinc, and after dinner his stomach pains led to his habitual dose of aluminum-containing antacids. His cognitive reserve was like a house on stilts hit by a tsunami. As his memory and emotional control began to leave him, you could almost see the neurons losing their grip on each other.

You want to prevent all of that. That means eating for excellent health, as we've seen in the preceding chapters. It also means using every opportunity to give your brain the stimulation it craves, whether that means a newspaper, a crossword puzzle, a class, or a news program. And why not go another step and jump into a challenging and fun online program, or see if a foreign language appeals to you? No matter what your age or past experience, you can find something you like.

By the way, Ben Pridmore is not the champion in all aspects

of memory. There is actually someone who can beat Ben. In Kyoto, Japan, researchers developed a computerized short-term memory test where Ben was resoundingly beaten. The computer program consisted of numbers that flashed momentarily in various places on a screen and were then suddenly replaced by blank squares.[9,10] The subject's task was to touch each square in what had been the correct numerical order. One, two, three, four, and so on.

Ben sidled up to the computer and did his very best. He was, in fact, very good. But Ben was resoundingly beaten by the local hero, Ayumu. And Ayumu was exactly seven years old at the time. His accuracy was far beyond anything Ben could approach.

Ayumu is a chimpanzee. In the laboratory of Dr. Tetsuro Matsuzawa, Ayumu competes against college students and anyone else who dares try. What Dr. Matsuzawa knows—and now all neuroscientists know—is that chimpanzees are much better than humans at memory tests like this, and no one beats Ayumu. It turns out that just as dogs detect smells and sounds that are out of humans' sensitivity range and starlings coordinate their flights millisecond by millisecond, chimpanzees have their own set of neuropsychological strengths that make us look like beginners.

If you'd like to try to beat Ayumu's average, Lumos Labs has prepared an online version of the test he is so good at. You'll see it at http://games.lumosity.com/chimp.html.

Of course, Ayumu has had a lot of practice, and figuring out what the humans around him are doing and saying has helped him build up a heck of a lot of cognitive reserve. Not to mention his diet. All those fruits and vegetables, with no meat, dairy products, or fatty foods, keep him fit, too.

CHAPTER 6

Physical Exercises That Protect Your Brain

Exercise is good for so many things, and brain health is one of them. As your heart starts pumping, you can just imagine the blood and oxygen surging to your brain, cleaning out the cobwebs and rejuvenating your brain cells. And it's true. People who exercise regularly have physical differences in their brains that can be seen on special brain scans. The hippocampus—the brain structure that is key for memory—is enhanced by any sort of exercise that gets your heart going. That appears to be true regardless of your age. And as the years go by, people who exercise are much less likely to develop Alzheimer's disease or have a stroke compared with their coach potato friends. Much as we might like to slip into a life of lazy leisure, the impressive power of exercise is going to lure us into breaking a sweat.

If you're not convinced, let me describe what science has shown:

Researchers at Columbia University invited a group of young

(twenty-one to forty-five years of age), out-of-shape volunteers to start an exercise program.[1] Everyone got his or her choice of a treadmill, bicycle, StairMaster, or elliptical trainer and was asked to exercise for forty minutes, four times a week for twelve weeks. The researchers then scanned their brains using magnetic resonance imaging (MRI). The scans indicated that their brains were actually building new blood vessels and new brain cells—not just anywhere but specifically in the hippocampus. The more physically fit the participants became, the more brain changes they had, and the stronger they performed on cognitive tests.

"But I'm not twenty-one years old!" you might be saying. Well, it looks like exercise works the same way—or even better— for older people. In fact, *it may actually reverse the gradual age-related shrinking of your brain.*

Researchers at the University of Illinois recruited fifty-nine adults—all were over age sixty and sedentary—for an exercise program.[2] Three times each week, the research volunteers got together for *aerobic* exercise, that is, activities designed to boost the heart rate (e.g., running, step exercises), as opposed to weight-lifting or stretching exercises that don't quicken your pulse.

After six months, the researchers measured the size of everyone's brains. Using MRI, they measured their gray matter—that is, the part of the brain made up mostly of brain cells (think of it as the business part of the brain). They also measured their white matter, which is made up mostly of *axons*—long wirelike processes extending from one brain cell to another. White matter is the collection of fibers that keep various parts of the brain and nervous system in communication with each other.

They then compared the results to MRIs done before the exercise program began. It turned out that after six months, the exercisers' gray matter was larger than before, especially in the frontal lobe areas essential for memory and attention. Their white matter was larger, too. The part of the white matter that had increased in size was the part of the brain that allows the right and left halves to communicate.

In a later study, researchers zeroed in on the *anterior hippocampus,* which typically shrinks about 1 to 2 percent per year as we age.[3] The researchers asked 120 older adults to start a simple walking program and tracked the size of the hippocampus in each person as the study went along.

Three times per week, the participants went for a walk. For the first week, the walks were just ten minutes long but were designed to be brisk enough that the participants' pulses noticeably increased. They then lengthened the walking sessions by five minutes each week, until they reached forty minutes in length. They then kept up the forty-minute walks and included five minutes of stretching before and after each walk.

MRI scans showed that, yes, exercise *reversed* the gradual brain shrinking that comes with age. That is, it increased the size of the anterior hippocampus. And, in the process, their memory performance improved, too.[3]

So does this mean that exercise might actually protect us against memory problems as we get older? In a word, yes. Researchers in Seattle's Group Health Cooperative found that among adults over age sixty-five, those who exercised three times a week were about 40 percent less likely to develop any sort of dementia compared with their not-so-active friends.[4] A five-year study in New York found much the same. People who exercised and followed a healthy diet cut their Alzheimer's risk by as much as 60 percent.[5]

Swedish researchers did the same kind of study—observing what happens to people as the years go by—and found that more physically active people were 60 percent less likely to develop Alzheimer's.[6] And *the benefit was especially noticeable among those with the APOE e4 gene,* suggesting once again that choices we make can override our genetic risks.

Several different research teams have estimated the benefit of exercise for preventing dementia, and although the benefits varied from one study to another, overall they show that regular aerobic exercise trims the risk of dementia by about 30 percent and cuts the risk of Alzheimer's disease roughly in half.[7]

How Does It Work?

Okay, so it works. But how? It is easy to see how running, biking, or tennis could strengthen your heart. But what exactly does exercise do to your brain? Well, for starters, exercise works in combination with a healthful diet to keep your arteries clear and open, maintaining a good blood supply. That means oxygen and nutrients go in and wastes come out. Exercise also helps you tackle blood pressure, diabetes, and weight problems, all of which affect the brain.

And part of the credit may go to a substance called BDNF, or *brain-derived neurotrophic factor,* which helps the brain grow new connections (synapses) between brain cells and protects the cells and connections you already have. Aerobic exercise increases the amount of BDNF in your brain.[3] That is important, because BDNF tends to be lower in people with Alzheimer's disease.

As your heart gets pumping, your brain starts laying down new connections between cells, and that seems to be true even for people with the APOE e4 gene.[7] Some researchers have also speculated that exercise helps your brain clear out toxins that could lead to the loss of brain cells.[8]

Think of what this means. Most people lose a bit of ground year by year. The connections from one cell to another start to fall away, and their brains shrink ever so slightly. As time goes on, they feel noticeably less sharp. But when you plug in the effect of regular heart-pumping exercise, everything starts to change. It is a bit like opening the garage door on your long-neglected Ferrari. You're dusting off your brain, blowing out the exhaust, and taking it out for a spin.

Your brain cells really are rejuvenated, and the results are clear on brain scans, in formal tests, and in how you feel from day to day.

Don't Wait

As I mentioned above, exercise is beneficial regardless of age. Even in preadolescence, children who are most physically fit do best on tests of cognitive function.[9] So whether you're twelve, forty-two, sixty-two, or ninety-two, exercises that get your pulse going are good for your brain.

Before You Begin

If the idea of beginning a new exercise program sounds a little daunting, let me reassure you. The program I am about to describe is easy. You'll go at your own pace. Before jumping in, let me mention a few important caveats:

Exercise along with a diet change, not instead of it. A bad diet can easily undo all the benefits of exercise. So be sure to follow the healthy diet steps described in the previous chapters. Give your Ferrari the fuel it needs.

The value of combining exercise with healthy eating applies not only to brain health but to physical health, as well. When people try to lose weight with exercise alone—without making any changes to what they are eating—they soon become disappointed.[10,11] To exercise away the calories in a six-piece order of chicken nuggets, you would have to run three miles. If you had a soda with it, that's another two and a half miles. If you had a burger at your next meal, that means three more miles. In theory, you could exercise all those calories away, but you would not have much time for anything else.

So let exercise add to the benefits of a healthy eating plan rather than take the place of it. As your healthy diet brings down your cholesterol level and helps you steer clear of toxic metals and other undesirables, your exercise regimen will enhance your benefits.

See your doctor. If you are over forty, have any health problems, or are significantly overweight, see your doctor before you start a new exercise program to make sure you are up to it. Your doctor can check your heart, joints, eyes, and feet.

He or she will also look over whatever medicines you may be taking. Some medicines will limit your ability to do aerobic exercise. For example, if you are on certain blood pressure medicines, your heartbeat will not respond as readily to exercise. So you'll want to be more cautious.

If you have diabetes, I have some special advice. If you have type 1 diabetes, your blood sugar can drop surprisingly quickly as you exercise. Ditto for people with type 2 diabetes who are taking medications, especially insulin or drugs that stimulate insulin secretion, such as glipizide, glyburide, glimepiride, nateglinide, or repaglinide. Sometimes the low blood sugar arrives quickly; other times it can be delayed for several hours. So you'll want to be ready for it. Carry a blood glucose monitor and glucose tablets for emergencies, and work with your health-care provider to adjust your eating schedule and medications if necessary.

Stay safe. There's a lot to be said for exercising with a partner, wearing good shoes, wrist protectors, and highly visible clothing, and staying away from traffic.

Start slowly. If you've been sedentary for some time, your body is not ready for a marathon. The arteries to your heart may have been narrowed by a not-so-healthy diet. Your joints are not ready for huge stresses either, and the last thing you want to do is to overwork your body. So take it easy at first. With time, you'll be able to do more and more. If you were to start a new swimming program, you wouldn't begin by crossing the English Channel. Any kind of aerobic exercise program should start well within your comfort zone.

Starting Your Exercise Program

Enough theory. It's time to get started. The program I am about to describe is based on walking. But rather than focusing on distance, we're going to focus on your pulse. The idea is to gently increase your pulse, boosting blood flow to the brain, for a prescribed period of time. And focusing on your pulse makes it really easy. You can walk and rest as much as you want to. There's never any need to be overly tired.

We'll begin by finding your zone—the pulse rate where you're getting benefits for your brain and body but are still within the bounds of safety. Then we'll gently pump up your pulse, getting the blood flowing to your brain. We'll gradually pick things up, letting you control the pace every step of the way. Finally, we'll take steps to keep you in the groove so that your exercise investment pays off maximally.

Find your target zone. As you exercise, you'll want to get your heart beating fast enough so that you benefit physically but not so fast that you strain your heart. To find the safety zone for your pulse rate, your doctor could give you a stress test. This is usually done by walking on a treadmill with wires from an electrocardiogram attached to your chest. The goal is to see how much you can exert yourself without signs of stress to the heart, such as chest pain or EKG changes.

A simpler way to calculate your safety zone is based on your age. First, subtract your age from 220. So, for example, if you are 60 years old, 220 minus 60 is 160. What you have just calculated is the absolute maximum pulse your heart could take. Now, for safety, you should stay well under that number.

Your target zone is between 60 percent and 80 percent of your maximal pulse. When you are starting out, aim for 60 percent of your maximum heart rate (for a sixty-year-old, that would be 96 beats per minute). When you are in better shape, you can push to 70 to 80 percent of your maximum heart rate—for a sixty-year-old, that would be 112 to 128 beats per minute. A highly trained athlete might push to 85 percent, but no one should go beyond that level. The table below will help you find your zone.

The idea of a target pulse zone is a welcome one for people who loathe the notion of jogging down the road for some interminable distance. Instead, you're just keeping your pulse up for a certain period of time. You can stop whenever you're uncomfortable and start again when you're ready.

Again, don't push it. Be sure to talk about your exercise plans with your doctor and follow his or her recommendations. It is important that you are comfortable as you exercise, can easily breathe and speak, and have no sensation of pain.

Find Your Zone

AGE	MAXIMUM PULSE	TARGET PULSE ZONE (60 TO 80%)
20	200	120–160
25	195	117–156
30	190	114–152
35	185	111–148
40	180	108–144
45	175	105–140
50	170	102–136
55	165	99–132
60	160	96–128
65	155	93–124
70	150	90–120
75	145	87–116
80	140	84–112
85	135	81–108
90	130	78–104
95	125	75–100
100	120	72–96

If you are in good shape now, a good way to begin is with a thirty-minute brisk walk three times per week. If you are not accustomed to brisk walking, you can start with just a ten-minute walk, and increase by five minutes each week. So during the first week, each walk lasts ten minutes. Feel free to walk more than once a day, but keep each walk within your limits. The second week, each walk lasts fifteen minutes, and so on until you reach forty or forty-five minutes. Then stay at that duration, with walks three or more times a week.

As you walk, you will want to let your pulse speed up,

assuming your doctor has not identified any reason not to do so. Your pulse should be higher than at rest and should be around your target zone. It should never be so fast that you cannot speak, have trouble breathing, or have any chest discomfort.

After a few minutes, check your pulse at your wrist or (gently) at your carotid artery, just to the side of your windpipe. Count the number of beats in fifteen seconds, and multiply by four to get the beats per minute.

Remember, you do not need to peg your workout to any certain distance. Rather, just aim to keep your heartbeat in your target zone for a period of time, as I described above. That means you can run, walk, or stop as much as you need to. The goal is to keep your pulse in the right zone. Before long you will find that you can sense whether your pulse is in the zone without actually checking it manually.

The Three Essentials

There are three keys to a successful exercise program:

Make it social. Some people go for the "no pain, no gain" mind-set and sign up for a boot camp experience where they get up at 5:30 in the morning to be yelled at by a former drill sergeant. But you are not one of them. Really, you won't stick with something unless you honestly enjoy it.

What turns physical activity into genuine fun is companionship. Go for a walk with a friend or family member. Pick a place you enjoy, whether that means natural surroundings, a busy urban avenue, or whatever your tastes call for.

If you join a gym, join with a friend if you can. And sign up for classes where you'll meet other people. We are much more likely to stick with an exercise plan if it's fun and if our companions are expecting us!

So take a minute now and think about how this can work for you. Who can you bring into your exercise routine? Where can you go to be with other people who are quickening their pulses, too?

By the way, exercise does not have to mean treadmills and weight lifting. It also means dancing, tennis, and a walk in the park. You can hold hands while you walk (particularly if you know each other).

Schedule it. To make it work, put it on your schedule—actually write it down. Things that get scheduled get done; things that are left to chance get neglected. Plan out your exercise program for the next three weeks, and treat it like a doctor's appointment or any other appointment you would be loath to miss.

So take a minute now and schedule it. Yes, actually jot it down on your calendar, and when exercise time comes up, off you go!

Keep it regular. Once you're in an exercise groove, it's easy to stay there. But if your exercise is only intermittent, your motivation really never gets off the couch. So keep it regular. If you set a rule that you're going for a brisk walk every day after dinner, or whatever schedule works for you, you'll find that you come to expect it and enjoy it. Don't let yourself have more than two sedentary days in a row.

Exercise is like an antibiotic. A single dose doesn't help very much. But if you take it on schedule, it's exactly the cure you're looking for.

So keep it social, put it on your schedule, and keep it regular, and everything else will fall into place.

Adding Variety

Go for variety. You might try a combination of walking and running. Or if you're feeling more energetic, go for bicycling, play tennis, go dancing, or whatever is your pleasure.

Don't disparage golf. Some people think of the sport as Mark Twain did—"a good walk ruined." I can't say I blame them. But if you can handle the humiliations of this challenging sport, you'll get a good walk in. Avoid the carts and especially avoid the foods served in the clubhouse.

Some people like exercise videos. They allow you to get hot and sweaty in the comfort of your own home. You'll find plenty of them online and at libraries.

You might like to use a pedometer. It's a little device clipped to your belt that tracks your steps. For some people, it brings in a bit of competitiveness in a good way. If they walked five thousand steps yesterday, they are going for seven thousand today. In our research studies, we use an Omron brand, but there are many others on the market. You can program in the length of your stride to track your mileage and how many calories you've burned. To give you a frame of reference, a vigorous day for a healthy, fit person would add up to about 10,000 steps. But stay within your own limits.

Whatever you do, don't let guilt invade your exercise life. Sometimes people scold themselves if they have not found the time to exercise. But it's really just a question of biology: Physical activity is good for us, and you can start when you're ready. And if you've drifted away from an exercise program, don't worry. It happens to everyone. Just dust yourself off and get back on when you can. Have fun with it.

Get All Three Kinds of Exercise

You'll want to tailor your exercise plan to your goals, thinking about the three different kinds of exercise, each of which has its own benefits:

Aerobic exercise means running, brisk walking, bicycling, an organized step-aerobic class, tennis, dancing, or any other continuous activity that gets your heart pumping. That's what we've focused on so far because, for brain protection, aerobic exercise is what really counts. This is the kind of exercise that boosts brain size and has been shown to noticeably improve working memory, planning, multitasking, and other cognitive functions.[12] It also improves your cardiac fitness, lowers your blood sugar and triglycerides, and reduces cancer risk. But there are two more kinds of exercise that will round out your benefits.

Resistance exercise builds muscular strength. Weight lifting, push-ups, and deep knee bends strengthen your skeleton, too. If your bone strength has been weakened by osteopenia or osteoporosis, working your muscles will, in turn, gradually strengthen your bones.

A typical regimen for resistance training works all major muscle groups three times a week. The workout would include three sets of eight to ten repetitions at a weight that cannot be lifted more than eight to ten times.

Flexibility exercises improve your joint range of motion, keep you limber, and help eliminate chronic pain. Yoga and Pilates are two excellent forms of flexibility exercises.

For resistance and flexibility training, I highly recommend having at least one session with a personal trainer. Everyone's needs and vulnerabilities differ so much that it really pays to have someone design a program that fits you.

If You Are Unable to Exercise

While I highly recommend exercise, some people cannot exercise to any meaningful degree due to a weak heart, joint problems, or severe obesity. If this includes you, you'll be glad to know that you can still benefit enormously from diet changes alone.

It might surprise you to learn that most of our research studies do not use exercise at all, because our goal is to see what diet changes alone can do. We are looking to test diet effects on weight, cholesterol, blood sugar, or other measures, and if people were to add exercise, it would confuse our tests. But we find that even when people do not change their exercise patterns, they still have enormous improvements in health. They lose weight, cholesterol and high blood pressure come down, and diabetes improves. Aches and pains start to melt away.

You may also find that after you begin a healthier way of eating, your heart becomes stronger, your joint pains start to disappear, your weight trims away, and you feel more energized. And then you may finally be able to exercise, perhaps for the first time in your life.

Born to Run?

Ever wonder why some people just love to exercise, while others find it daunting? It's not a question of character. It's biology.

Some people are born with muscles that have a great many "type I" cells—special muscle cells that have a rich supply of capillaries to bring in oxygen, remove waste products, and prevent fatigue. These cells also have a large quantity of an enzyme called lipoprotein lipase, which breaks fats apart to be used as fuel. If your muscles are loaded with type I cells, you'll feel like running long after your friends have collapsed from exhaustion.

Type II cells are different. They are fine for a short sprint, but they run out of gas before you've gone very far.

So when people love exercise or loathe it, it's mostly a question of biology—the kind of muscle cells they were born with.

But here's what counts: *You can change the makeup of your muscles.* With vigorous exercise, type II cells start to get a better and better blood supply, eventually making them very much like type I cells.

Exercise aptitude is largely genetic, but exercise itself can compensate for what nature might have forgotten.

Extra Benefits

So exercise counters brain shrinking and helps everything work better. It also has some important "side effects." First, the physical ones:

- Exercise helps you lose weight. It adds to your overall calorie burn, and is also calorie-free. You just can't dip shrimp into tartar sauce while you're playing tennis, and it's hard to scarf down a burger on your bicycle.
- For your heart, exercise improves cardiac fitness, reduces blood pressure, boosts HDL ("good") cholesterol, and trims triglycerides.
- Women who exercise have less risk of developing breast cancer and better survival if cancer strikes.

There are some big psychological benefits, too:

- Physical activity helps you sleep better. It's not hard to see why: As your muscles become tired, they demand sleep. And when you've slept well, you feel like sticking to a healthier lifestyle. Moreover, sleep might even help you prevent Alzheimer's disease, as we will see in the next chapter.

• Exercise is a natural antidepressant. In some studies, it is about as effective as antidepressant medications.

Fueling Your Exercise

Let me repeat a key point: *It is essential to exercise along with a healthy diet, not in place of it.* So many people imagine that because they have exercised, they can dig into unhealthy foods. But exercise cannot "burn off" cholesterol, and it is a lot to ask for exercise to undo the effects of a bad diet.

Think of physical exercise as an important tool in your toolbox. Start with a healthy diet, add mental and physical exercises, and you're taking real power into your hands.

Step III

DEFEAT MEMORY THREATS

By now you've learned a great deal about how nutrients protect your brain and how exercises—physical and mental—strengthen your neural connections and reverse age-related brain shrinkage. But, as important as they are, these steps can be defeated if you do not avert certain common memory threats.

Sleep is when memories are consolidated, like files being neatly stored in a filing cabinet. If your sleep is disturbed, your memory "files" remain in a jumble, and you'll have trouble coming up with names and words you need.

In addition, certain medications and health conditions can wreak havoc with your brain cells. Many people have no idea that their memory problems can be solved simply by changing a prescription or correcting an underlying medical condition.

Let me encourage you not only to read through the following chapters carefully, but also to take this book with you when you see your physician. You can use it as a checklist for medicines and medical conditions that may merit investigation.

CHAPTER 7

Build Memory Power as You Sleep

When I entered my third year of medical school, I quickly learned how important sleep is for memory. The year started out on the surgical wards of the George Washington University Hospital, and the schedule was punishing. The workweek started at 8 a.m. on Monday. We worked all day Monday, Monday night, and all day Tuesday, before finally going home Tuesday evening—a shift lasting more than thirty-two hours at a stretch. Then Wednesday was a normal workday of eight or ten hours. On Thursday it started again—working all day Thursday, Thursday night, and Friday, before collapsing at home on Friday night. We worked weekends, too. The schedule went on and on, seven days a week. Students, interns, residents—we all lived that way.

Reading this, you are no doubt horrified that clinical care would be in the hands of chronically sleep-deprived people. Luckily, things have changed a lot since then.

After just a few days on this schedule, I discovered that my short-term memory had become a sieve. Medication orders I had to write, patients I needed to see, lab results that needed to be checked—unless I wrote down *everything,* it all tended to slip away. The other medical trainees experienced exactly the same thing. With long sleepless stretches, our memory capacity was shot. Then, when we finally got a vacation and started to catch up on sleep, our memories returned to normal.

Sleep is important. As you doze off to sleep and your brain no longer has to pay attention to your conscious life, it can file away the experiences of the day, reset your emotional balance, shore up your pain control, and generally tidy up. At night, your brain is like a road crew that comes out on the highway after dark, setting out orange cones, filling potholes, painting lines, repaving, and then disappearing before the morning rush hour begins. If you keep going twenty-four hours a day, your potholes never get a chance to be filled in.

If it surprises you that your brain needs rest, think about all the other parts of your body. You can't push your muscles twenty-four hours a day. After physical exercise, they need rest in order to repair and recharge. Every athlete knows that giving your muscles and joints time to recover and rebuild after exercise is as important as exercise itself.

Brain researchers say that sleep helps the brain *consolidate* memories. Let's say that you've learned some new facts from a book or perhaps you gained some new skills on a musical instrument. Those memory traces are fragile at first and can easily be lost. Sleep helps them become permanent.

Research suggests that the first half of the night is when we consolidate memories of facts and events. The second half of the night, when rapid eye movement (REM) sleep is more predominant, is when we integrate memories related to new skills and to emotions.[1]

In the first part of the night, your body greatly reduces its production of *cortisol*. Cortisol is a hormone best known for its role in stress. It signals you to be alert to dangers and gets you ready for fight or flight. And when your brain is trying to file things away, the last thing it needs is to be distracted with a cortisol-driven high alert. So your brain turns down the cortisol and gets on with the work at hand.

In experiments, researchers have infused cortisol intrave-nously in sleeping human volunteers during the early part of the night and have found that it severely reduces their ability to retain memories for facts and events.[1]

So a medical student who, at one o'clock in the morning, is drawing a blood sample from a patient, then running the blood tubes to the laboratory, then wheeling a patient from the emer-gency room to a hospital bed, then consoling the family of a trauma victim and doing all the things medical students do is not only neglecting his or her need for sleep. That student is under stress, which stimulates the release of cortisol—the very hormone that interferes with memory consolidation when the brain is asleep. Even if the student could take a few minutes to doze off while the lab runs a test or a patient is having an X-ray, that sleep will not be of much use.

It is not just medical students who have this problem. Accountants, teachers, truck drivers, overworked parents, fac-tory workers on swing shifts, members of Congress, and just about everyone else is prone to burning their candles at both ends, boosting their cortisol levels and interfering with memory.

In the second half of the night, everything changes. Rapid eye movement is a sign that you are dreaming. The facts and details that were important in the first half of the night now give way to the absurd dramas of dreams, infused with emotions of all kinds. And now cortisol levels start to rise. Some have suggested that just as cortisol interferes with memory consolidation early in sleep, it also softens emotional memories later in the night, so they are less intense and more manageable.

People with post-traumatic stress disorder get none of the softening of unpleasant memories that most of us thankfully experience. They repeatedly reexperience terrifying memories of traumatic events. Blood tests show that for some reason, they do not get the same cortisol rise that other people get in the second half of the night.[1]

Sleep and Amyloid

Sleep may play an even bigger role in preserving your memory, a research team at Washington University in St. Louis has found. The researchers collected the cerebrospinal fluid from volunteers, using tiny tubes passed into their lower backs.[2] Every hour for thirty-six hours, the researchers took a small sample while the volunteers talked, watched television, ate, or slept. What they were looking for was amyloid.

As you know well by now, the microscopic amyloid plaques that develop in the brain have been under intense study by researchers who are trying to understand why they form and how they contribute to memory loss. Amyloid is produced by brain cells, and eventually it flows down the spinal column, which is where the researchers were able to measure it.

The research team noticed several important things. First of all, amyloid has a circadian rhythm. That is, it rises and falls like a tide, day after day. A surge in amyloid production is followed by a prolonged lull, and then the cycle begins again, day after day.

The question, then, is what drives this cycle? If we could find out what causes the ebb and flow of amyloid, maybe we could have less of it, and reduce the brain-damaging effects it seems to have.

Maybe amyloid production rises at mealtime. Or maybe it's physical activity that causes a rise in amyloid that then slacks off when we settle down. Or perhaps it's just a day-night cycle, as is the case for many other hormones.

So the St. Louis researchers set up video cameras to watch what people were doing and simultaneously measured the amyloid in their cerebrospinal fluid. They watched them eating, talking, reading, sleeping, watching television, typing on their computers, and even using the bathroom. They tracked their body positions—flat, upright, or in between. And they looked at whether the amount of amyloid in their cerebrospinal fluid rose or fell with each activity.

Here is what they found: It did not matter if people were sitting, standing, or lying down. It did not matter if they were quietly reading, as opposed to walking around the room. It did not make much difference if they were sitting with their eyes closed versus having their brains get intensive stimulation from a television program or video game.

What mattered was whether they were awake. Amyloid goes up while you are awake and it falls when you go to sleep. The research team speculated that during sleep, the brain is able to clear itself of amyloid.

So this suggests that you have some control over your brain's amyloid production. If you're burning the midnight oil over a work project, watching the late show, or having a late-night snack, your brain stays up with you, cranking out amyloid all the while, or so it seems. If instead you go to sleep, your amyloid factories can finally turn out the lights, too. The sooner you go to sleep, the quicker they can close down. Sleep helps you shut off amyloid.

The St. Louis team noticed something else. Sleep seems less effective at shutting off amyloid production in older people compared with younger people. But the benefit of sleep never seems to be gone. The moral of the story is that sleep deprivation is among the worst things you can inflict on your brain. Those neurons are eager for you to get plenty of shut-eye.

As you read this text, please look up and check the clock. If it is after 10 p.m., close this book and go to bed. Your brain is tired, and you need to stop pushing it to create amyloid.

The Other Advantage of Being Unconscious

Sleep brings you one more benefit. When you're unconscious, you can't reach for a doughnut. And, yes, people who turn out the light and go to sleep early are thinner than people who stay up late. That's good for your waistline, and, in turn, a trim waistline is good for health overall and for brain health in particular.

Getting a Good Night's Sleep

Sleep is your brain's best friend. But many people have trouble getting a good night's sleep. They lie down but just can't seem to doze off. Or they wake up early, unable to return to sleep. Or perhaps they don't give themselves the chance to sleep, staying awake till all hours, and setting the alarm to go off long before they have had a full night's sleep.

If sleep is a challenge for you, let me offer some important tips, starting with a look at a few seemingly innocuous things that can be sleep destroyers:

Caffeine. If caffeine does not interfere with your sleep, you feel mentally fine, and your memory is sharp, don't worry about it. The health issues related to caffeine are pretty minor. In fact, some evidence suggests that vigorous coffee drinkers actually have less risk of Alzheimer's disease, as we saw in chapter 4. But if you're tossing and turning, it is time to own up to what caffeine does.

In a word, it persists. If you have a cup of coffee at 8 a.m., a quarter of its caffeine is still circulating in your bloodstream at 8 p.m.

If you like technical explanations, the *half-life* of caffeine—the time it takes for your body to eliminate half the caffeine in your bloodstream—is about six hours. So the caffeine in your 8 a.m. cup of coffee is half gone by 2 p.m., and three-quarters gone by 8 p.m. But that remaining quarter-cup's worth of caffeine can be enough to keep you from sliding into a deep and restful sleep.

And, worse, electroencephalograph (EEG) tests show that caffeine decreases the slow-wave sleep that is essential for memory consolidation in the early part of the night. So you might learn all kinds of things during the day, only to have them vanish in the night, as caffeine prevents your brain from making these fragile traces permanent.

"But I feel *better* when I have a cup of coffee," you say. "And I feel terrible without it." Of course you do. Many coffee drinkers feel very much that way. But caffeine is a complex drug. First of all, it is a mild painkiller, which is why it is added to many over-the-counter analgesics. It is also a stimulant. When your brain is habituated to these effects, you really will feel horrible when you miss your dose. You are in withdrawal.

And caffeine's effects on your mental clarity are something else. It may help you stay awake and may take the edge off your aches and pains, but that does not mean your thinking is clear, your emotions are balanced, or your outlook is bright. For some people, caffeine keeps them awake, but mentally dull, fuzzy, or on edge.

Now, everyone is different. Some people metabolize caffeine more quickly, while others eliminate it more slowly. It pays to notice how caffeine affects you.

If you do break a caffeine habit, you may notice that your thinking becomes noticeably clearer, your personality becomes brighter and more flexible, irritability subsides, and the world feels like a better place to live. Before you get there, you will go through a few days of withdrawal as caffeine makes its last fading pleas for your loyalty, but you'll very likely be glad you left it behind.

Alcohol. Alcohol is a bit of a devil. A drink or two gently lulls you to sleep. But in the early morning hours, your sleep starts to lighten. Around 4 a.m., worries wake you up, and you find yourself poring over problems left over from the previous day.

This early-morning awakening is not caused by mixing red wine with white or by the sediment in dark beer. It is caused by alcohol molecules transforming into closely related chemicals, called aldehydes. They are stimulants. These maladjusted chemicals have none of alcohol's charms and instead make your sleep rocky.

Protein. Protein in the morning helps you stay alert. It does this by blocking your brain's ability to produce serotonin, the mood-regulating chemical that also helps you sleep. So if your breakfast included some beans or soy products, such as veggie sausage, veggie bacon, or scrambled tofu, you'll feel noticeably more alert than if you just had, say, a bagel. If you have your high-protein food first, and a starchier food second, you'll be fine. Notice that I have mentioned vegetarian versions of high-protein foods. You do not want to do yourself the harm of including bacon, sausage, eggs, or other fatty, high-cholesterol foods in your routine.

At night, you want the opposite effect. That is, you want your brain to make serotonin to help you calm down and go to sleep. So let your dinner include more starches, and avoid high-protein foods. Natural starches, such as rice, pasta, and bread, stimulate serotonin production in your brain. You'll find it easier to doze off and to stay asleep.

Foods and Serotonin

Protein blocks serotonin production in your brain, while carbohydrate has the opposite effect, helping you make serotonin. That's important, because serotonin helps you sleep. Here's how:

A protein molecule is like a string of beads. Each bead is an *amino acid.* When you digest protein, the string breaks apart and each "bead"—that is, each amino acid—passes from your digestive tract into your bloodstream. One particular amino acid, called *tryptophan*, then passes from your bloodstream into your brain, where it turns into serotonin.

However, if you have a high-protein meal, it sends a great many amino acids into your bloodstream. And the more of them there are in your blood, the harder it is for tryptophan to work its way through the crowd and get into your brain. There is just too much competition from all those other amino acids. So even though high-protein foods contain some tryptophan, they have many other amino acids that compete with it. The net effect is that tryptophan is crowded out of the brain. Your brain ends up with *less* serotonin.

At night, you *want* tryptophan to get into your brain so it can make serotonin that can help you sleep. The answer is carbohydrates. Starchy foods stimulate the release of insulin, which removes many of the competing amino acids from the bloodstream, leaving tryptophan behind to circulate freely in the blood. Tryptophan then easily passes into the brain and produces serotonin, which helps you sleep.

So a starchy food can be a natural sleeping pill. But if you want to stay alert, high-protein foods, such as beans or tofu, are your best choices.

The call of the bathroom. If you're getting up several times a night for a trip to the bathroom, you're interrupting your brain's nighttime routine. It might pay to drink a bit less water in the evening.

If those seductive bubbles in your sparkling water are making you drink more than you need, your body soaks that water up like a sponge, only to release it later on. Switch to still water and you'll be less likely to overdo it.

You also may benefit from cutting down on salty foods. Salt holds water in your bloodstream and body tissues, and as the night progresses, that water gradually finds its way through your kidneys and into your bladder, waking you up.

If you're in the bathroom several times a night because of prostate problems, it's time for a good medical evaluation and perhaps treatment. And some evidence suggests that a plant-based diet—the same one that is good for your heart and helps prevent strokes and Alzheimer's disease—is good for your prostate, too.

Lack of exercise. If you have plenty of physical activity during the day, you will sleep better at night. Think about children. They run around so much all day that they are practically comatose at night. As we get older, we tend to be less physically active. For some of us, the only exercise we get is the tips of our fingers typing on a keyboard. So when we lie down to sleep, our brains might feel tired, but our muscles are not, so they do not demand sleep. Your sleep will then be light and easily interrupted by the slightest noise or worry. And you will end up dragging through the day.

So to get a good night's sleep, get a little exercise. The best exercises for a good night's sleep are those that put a bit of strain on your muscles—push-ups or weight lifting, for example. Even a little exercise can have a noticeable effect on sleep.

It goes without saying that you should talk with your doctor before starting a new exercise program. You'll want to be sure your heart and joints, in particular, are ready for it.

A pre-bedtime routine. If you have a cat, watch what your cat does before going to sleep. She'll stretch out her paws, give a big yawn, and then curl up and go to sleep. Dogs do the same. In medical school, I had a pet rat who'd been saved from a laboratory, and she used to stretch out her cute little rat paw, give a yawn, and dream about trigonometry or the rings of Saturn, or whatever rats dream about.

People do the same. Children stretch and yawn, getting ready for sleep. But have you noticed that adults often do not go through this ritual? Whether it is due to caffeine, stress, or something else, they simply close their magazine, turn out the light, and hope to doze off.

If you had imagined that these presleep rituals have no function, try a little test. About a half-hour before bedtime, open your mouth to simulate a big yawn. Reach out your arms and give them a good stretch. At first you're just going through the motions. But do this four times—a big yawn and a stretch each time. You'll soon trigger a genuine yawn and a deep-muscle stretch. Then notice what this does to the quality of the sleep that follows. What you will likely discover is that something about stretching and yawning prepares the body and brain for sleep.

If you are having trouble sleeping, use this simple routine, and see if it helps.

Nap If You Need It

Some people are afraid to nap during the day for fear they won't sleep at night. That's possible, if it is a very long nap. But a short nap will not interfere with sleep and might actually help you get rid of accumulated tension so you'll unwind more easily at night.

A Word About Sleep Medications

A man in Virginia woke up to the sound of his alarm and went down to the kitchen to fix his breakfast. And there on the kitchen table was an open box of cereal, a selection of fruit, a loaf of bread, and a variety of other groceries. "That's strange," he thought. "Who put those there?" He looked in his refrigerator and found it surprisingly well stocked with orange juice, cartons of almond milk, salad ingredients, and many other things. Since he lived alone, these magically appearing groceries were a puzzle.

The night before, he had taken zolpidem, the massively popular sleeping pill, marketed under the name Ambien. Under its influence, he had driven to the store and stocked up for the week, and all memories of the shopping trip were wiped out before morning. Many other people have reported similar bizarre experiences of sleepwalking, sleep-driving, or binge-eating, with subsequent amnesia for the impromptu party they had put on for themselves the night before.

Some sleep experts swear by Ambien, saying it is much safer than many older sleep aids. But the fact is, memory problems are very common, and Ambien's prescribing information has been updated to include stern warnings about people doing all sorts of other things they cannot remember later. I strongly suggest you avoid it.

Other sleeping medications can affect memory, too. Some of them block the neurotransmitter *acetylcholine*. On this list are diphenhydramine (Benadryl, Sominex) and doxylamine, which is found not only in sleeping medications (such as Unisom) but also in nighttime cold remedies (such as NyQuil, Alka-Seltzer Plus Night Cold, and Tylenol Flu Nighttime). If you block acetyl-choline too strongly—for example by taking too large of a dose or by combining two or more medicines with similar effects—you can end up with dry mouth, blurred vision, constipation, urinary retention, and, eventually, confusion and memory problems.

Many antidepressants are used for sleep, too, and their tendency to block acetylcholine can cause the same problem. We'll have more to say about medications in chapter 8.

Wealthy and Wise

Sleep is essential for memory and many other aspects of health. I would encourage you to turn out the lights at 10 p.m. and let your brain get on with the work of repairing and rebuilding.

Be careful about caffeine and alcohol, skip high-protein foods late in the day, get plenty of exercise, and try the pre-sleep routines I mentioned. Your brain will thank you for it.

CHAPTER 8

Medicines and Health Conditions That Affect Memory

A man walks out of the clinic, where he just had a routine colonoscopy. "The doctor says I'm fine," he tells his wife who is waiting in the car. "He doesn't need to see me for another five years."

"Wonderful!" she says. "Did it hurt?"

"Ummm, well..." he stammers. "Actually, I don't know. I don't remember a thing about it. It's weird—I can't remember anything."

The reason he doesn't remember is that his doctors slipped him a dose of a drug that wiped out his memory of the event. Called midazolam and marketed under the brand name Versed (pronounced *ver-SEDD*), the drug is routinely used after minor surgical procedures. The colonoscopy could have been smooth as silk or excruciatingly uncomfortable—the medical team could have danced on the table and sung "Auld Lang Syne"—and the patient, who had been wide awake the whole time, would not remember one jot of it. While patients might well object to the idea of being given a drug to wipe out their memory banks, the practice is as routine as hand-washing.

I once asked a colonoscopy nurse why they always used Versed. "So patients will come back," she said. If patients remembered every last discomfort and indignity of the procedure, they would be a lot less eager for their next exam. Some anesthesiologists use propofol (marketed as Diprivan) rather than Versed. Propofol was the drug that, in combination with other drugs, was implicated in Michael Jackson's death. It causes a similar amnesia.

Versed is an extreme illustration of an important fact: Drugs can wreak havoc with your memory. Versed is in the same chemical class as Valium, Ativan, and Xanax—all of which are commonly used for anxiety. They can all affect memory, albeit not so decisively as Versed.

And so can many other medications. Even common cholesterol-lowering drugs, including Lipitor and Crestor, can cause memory deficits that mimic early Alzheimer's disease. You discover the truth only when you stop the medication and find that your memory gradually returns.

But there is an even more fundamental point: *All kinds of things* can affect your memory. A great many medical conditions can cloud your thinking. As words start escaping you and you start to feel less and less like yourself, there may well be a simple reason that can be identified and fixed.

In this chapter, we'll look at the conditions that can harm your memory and what you can do about them.

Medicines That Muddle Memory

When anyone experiences any sort of memory problem, medications should be high on the list of suspects. Unfortunately, many people, including many doctors, do not think to look there until problems have carried on too long. Below we will look at specific medications that interfere with memory or cause other cognitive problems. But first, a few important points:

• **Medication effects add up.** The effects of one medication can add to those of another. For example, you might be taking an antidepressant that blocks a brain chemical called *acetylcholine*. Aside from a little dry mouth or constipation, the side effects are not too bad. But then later on you might need an allergy medicine, and it blocks *acetylcholine*, too. With two drugs blocking the same brain chemical, their side effects add up, and it can be too much for the brain, clouding your thinking and interfering with memory. A common scenario is that one doctor prescribes a medication. Then another doctor prescribes a second medicine for an unrelated condition. More and more drugs are added, but none of the doctors look at the full list of pharmaceuticals marinating the patient's brain. Medicines, of course, are very useful and sometimes lifesaving. But it is important to step back from time to time and take a fresh look at what you are taking.

• **Drugs can interact with food.** If you were to sip a grapefruit juice, you probably wouldn't imagine that it could disable the enzymes your liver uses to break down Versed and Lipitor. But it does, and that means the drugs stay in your blood much longer, heightening their assault on your memory. Grapefruit juice has a similar effect for many other medicines, too, typically lasting for about twenty-four hours after your last glass of juice.

• **Talk with your doctor—now.** If you suspect that medications may be causing a problem, speak with your doctor. It is often possible to discontinue one or more medications to see if memory improves. However, the safety of taking a "medication vacation" and how to go about it differ from medicine to medicine. For example, there is little risk to stopping a cholesterol-lowering drug such as atorvastatin (Lipitor) for a few months, but stopping a blood pressure medication could lead to a prompt and dangerous increase in your blood pressure. Ditto for diabetes medicines; stopping them could mean a risky spike in your blood sugar. You do not want to stop them on your own. Also, stopping some medications can lead to withdrawal symptoms. Anxiety medications, for example, can be habituating, and it can be dangerous to stop them abruptly. The answer, in every case, is to speak with your doctor before making any changes in your medications.

• **Keep a list.** It pays to keep a list of any medications you are taking. Update it regularly, and give a copy to any doctor you happen to consult. Include the drug name, size of each pill (milligrams), what time of day you take it, and the number of pills you take each time. This will make your doctor's job easy and will help prevent mistakes.

Here are the most common culprits—medications that are known to cause cognitive problems. This does not mean that they *always* cause problems—for some medications, memory problems are quite uncommon—or that they can be blamed for cognitive problems in any given person. But when you are looking for answers, these medications should be on your list of suspects.

Cholesterol-lowering drugs. Cholesterol-lowering drugs are among the most commonly prescribed medications. With well over $10 billion in annual sales, Lipitor was the world's leading pharmaceutical moneymaker before going generic in 2011.

Lipitor is a *statin*, the group that also includes Crestor, Mevacor, Zocor, and many others. Generally, their safety profile is good. In fact, lowering cholesterol is one way to reduce the risk of Alzheimer's disease and stroke. Because statins are so widely prescribed, many people imagine they are innocuous. Some doctors refer to Lipitor as "vitamin L," and some have even suggested it be sold without a prescription, like aspirin or vitamins.

However, statins do have side effects, some of which are serious. They can cause muscle and liver toxicity and, in high doses, are linked to diabetes.[1] And a number of people have reported striking effects on their memory: confusion, disorientation, and memory gaps that look like the beginnings of Alzheimer's disease.

Duane Graveline is a physician and a former NASA astronaut who lives near the Kennedy Space Center on Florida's Atlantic coast. Returning home from a walk one day, he felt totally disoriented. He had no idea where he was. A woman came out to greet him, and he did not recognize her. This was his wife, who saw that something was very wrong with Duane. His memory banks had been wiped out. Later on in the hospital emergency room, he tried to piece things together. The only explanation he could think of for his bizarre amnesia was the Lipitor he had started several weeks earlier. Stopping the medicine cured his memory loss.

But later on, he restarted Lipitor at half the dose, only to find that, after about six weeks, it scuttled his memory again, erasing everything after high school, including his wife, children, and everyone else. He looked into the effects of statins on memory and ended up dedicating several books (*The Dark Side of Statins* and *Statin Drugs: Side Effects and the Misguided War on*

Cholesterol, among others) and a website (www.SpaceDoc.com) to getting the word out.

At the University of California at San Diego, Beatrice Golomb documented 171 cases of people who reported significant cognitive problems while taking statins.[2] In 90 percent of cases, stopping the drug fixed the problem, often within days. Some of these people had been mistakenly diagnosed with Alzheimer's disease—diagnoses that no longer applied. Some later resumed taking statins—sometimes several times—only to find their symptoms returning each time. The higher the dose, the more likely they were to have problems, and some people have not fully recovered, even years after stopping the medication.

The side effect seems to be uncommon. But with so many people taking statins, even rare side effects mount up. And doctors treating older people may mistakenly assume that their symptoms are age-related or are attributable to Alzheimer's disease, and may never stop the drug to see if things clear up.

Luckily, there are other ways to lower your cholesterol, as we saw in chapter 3. A chicken-and-fish diet is not very effective, but when people set aside animal products and greasy foods altogether, the effect on their cholesterol levels can be so dramatic that medications are usually unnecessary.

COMMONLY PRESCRIBED CHOLESTEROL-LOWERING STATIN DRUGS

Brand names are in parentheses:

atorvastatin (Lipitor)

ezetimibe/simvastatin (Vytorin)

fluvastatin (Lescol)

lovastatin (Mevacor)

pravastatin (Pravachol)

rosuvastatin (Crestor)

simvastatin (Zocor)

Sleep medications. In the preceding chapter I mentioned the surprising memory problems that can come from sleeping pills. I strongly suggest avoiding sleeping medications, if possible, and using the more natural approaches to sleep that I described. Common sleeping medications that can interfere with memory include:

diphenhydramine (Benadryl, Sominex)

doxylamine (Unisom, NyQuil, Alka-Seltzer Plus Night Cold, Tylenol Flu Nighttime)

zolpidem (Ambien)

Antidepressants. Antidepressants work by changing the balance of neurotransmitters that control moods. Some also block acetylcholine, so confusion and memory problems can occasionally occur.

Antidepressants for which memory effects have been commonly reported are listed below.

amitriptyline (Elavil)

desipramine (Norpramin)

imipramine (Tofranil)

nortriptyline (Pamelor)

venlafaxine (Effexor)

Keep in mind, however, that *any* antidepressant can be considered a possible contributor to confusion or memory problems. Even antidepressants that have little or no effect on acetylcholine—fluoxetine (Prozac) and paroxetine (Paxil), for example—should be considered suspects if clouded thinking or memory problems arise.

Many people are tackling depression by other means altogether, often with spectacular results. New psychotherapy methods are much quicker than previous treatments and work very well. Exercise has also been shown to lift moods, perhaps as well as antidepressant drugs. Of course, if you're depressed, you may not feel like exercising—or doing much of anything—but once you start, you find that you get an energy boost, and the noticeable payoff keeps you going.

Antihistamines. Many allergy pills block acetylcholine, the neurotransmitter mentioned above. With occasional use, this is not likely to be a problem, but if you take these medications over extended periods or take more than one medication with this same action, side effects are more likely. Common antihistamines in this category include:

brompheniramine (such as Dimetapp)
chlorpheniramine (such as Chlor-Trimeton)
clemastine (such as Tavist)
diphenhydramine (such as Benadryl)

Newer antihistamines, such as fexofenadine (Allegra) and cetirizine (Zyrtec), are less likely to have these undesirable effects.

Anxiety medications. Valium, Ativan, Xanax, and other popular anxiety medications are in the same chemical class as Versed, the operating-room drug I mentioned at the beginning of this chapter. They do not have anywhere near its power to erase memories. But they can nonetheless impair your memory and blunt your emotions.

It is important to be aware that anxiety drugs are clumsy. When they reach into your brain, they do more than simply turn down the anxiety button. They bump into many different parts of the brain and adjust brain chemistry in myriad ways, not all of which are helpful.

One more problem: With prolonged use, you can become physically dependent on anxiety drugs, as I mentioned above. This does not mean that you will end up in a back alley buying your next dose, but it does mean that stopping them abruptly can lead to rebound anxiety and even seizures. To prevent this, your doctor will taper you off gradually.

COMMON ANXIETY MEDICATIONS

alprazolam (Xanax)
clonazepam (Klonopin)
diazepam (Valium)
lorazepam (Ativan)
oxazepam (Serax)
temazepam (Restoril)
triazolam (Halcion)

Painkillers. Many people take analgesics on a daily basis for chronic pain. Opiate pain relievers (such as morphine, oxycodone, and hydrocodone) can interfere with your memory over the short term, although most people who take them on a more ongoing basis for chronic pain seem to habituate to their effects and do not have serious cognitive problems.[3] Even so, if you are on painkillers and having memory problems, it is worth speaking to your physician about alternatives to your current medications.

If you are using pain medications for rheumatoid arthritis, migraines, or fibromyalgia, let me encourage you to see if a dietary approach might help. Many people find that these painful conditions are triggered by specific foods, such as dairy products, eggs, white potatoes, and a short list of others. In a previous book, *Foods That Fight Pain,* I detailed a simple way to sort out whether eliminating one or more of these foods can cure your problem.

142   POWER FOODS FOR THE BRAIN

Do not take this on faith. You might simply give it a try and see for yourself. Not everyone finds a food trigger, but when you do, a diet adjustment can allow you to reduce or eliminate your need for medication.

Blood pressure medicines. Blood pressure medicines have been shown to affect memory in rare cases. Propranolol is sometimes used to reduce blood pressure and more often to slow a rapid heart beat (tachycardia). It can affect the brain.

However, high blood pressure is dangerous and is a key contributor to stroke risk. So if you are on a blood pressure medication, be sure to speak with your doctor before changing the dose.

At the same time, do not neglect nondrug methods that can improve your blood pressure. Weight loss, limiting sodium, following a plant-based diet, and exercise can go a long way toward eliminating the need for blood pressure drugs. See chapter 4 for more details on how diet changes can help.

Acid blockers. Many people use medications to block the production of stomach acid. Ranitidine (Zantac) and cimetidine (Tagamet) have been reported to cause confusion in rare cases. Luckily, the problem disappears when the medication is stopped.

Our Drug Culture

The medicines listed above are the common offenders. But other drugs could affect memory, too, and new ones enter the market every year. Often their full range of side effects does not become clear for several years.

The problem is likely to get worse before it gets better. In recent years, drugmakers have realized that they do not make much money from medicines that are used for just a few days or weeks at a time, such as antibiotics. So they are investing heavily in medicines that are used essentially for life. Cholesterol drugs, diabetes drugs, blood pressure drugs, and arthritis drugs are the pharmaceutical industry's little golden eggs.

The Food and Drug Administration does not require Lipitor's manufacturer to disclose to patients that many of them would not need the drug at all if they were to follow a plant-based diet. Nor does it require manufacturers of diabetes or blood pressure medicines to reveal that similar menu changes would reduce the need for those drugs, too. On the contrary, drug companies spend a fortune "educating" us about the essential nature of their products. Their continuing medical education courses for doctors, grants to medical centers, and prime-time television advertisements are all designed to help us forget that many of our most common medical problems have their roots in diet and lifestyle.

So do take advantage of the benefits of medicines when you need them. But be cautious, and always be alert to the possibility of side effects, especially if the number of medications you take increases.

Hidden Medical Problems

If you are experiencing memory problems, you will want to speak with your doctor about possible hidden causes. Here are some important ones to consider:

Gluten Intolerance

Could your choice of bread affect your brain? If you're gluten intolerant, it could. Gluten is a protein found in wheat, barley, and rye. For most people, it is easy to digest and is healthful and nutritious. But about 1 percent of people have a hereditary condition called celiac disease. If you are one of them, your body will react to gluten like a toxin. It can damage your intestinal tract, causing diarrhea and other digestive symptoms.

In the mid-1990s, researchers realized that problems go further. Many people with celiac disease find that even small amounts of these problem grains cause fatigue and mental fuzziness. The good news is that by avoiding gluten, the symptoms vanish.

Testing for celiac disease is easy. Your doctor simply draws a blood sample to check for the antibodies that are the hallmark of the condition. If it looks like you have it, your doctor may perform a small bowel biopsy to check for damage. However, if you suspect you have a gluten problem, you can easily just go gluten-free for a few weeks without testing to see if your symptoms resolve. Let me hasten to add that if you are not sensitive to gluten (the vast majority of people are not), there is no health reason to avoid it.

If you would like to see what a gluten-free diet can do for you, simply avoid wheat, barley, and rye. You should have no problem with rice, corn, millet, quinoa, amaranth, or buckwheat; and vegetables, fruits, beans, tofu, and so on should be fine, too. But you'll have to read labels, because if you have celiac disease, even the slightest trace of gluten, like the wheat in soy sauce or the barley in a canned soup, will cause a reaction.

Oats do not contain gluten, so in theory they should be okay. Unfortunately, some oat products harbor traces of other grains, which has led some companies (such as Bob's Red Mill) to use special production facilities that prevent cross-contamination. You may find it prudent to strike oats off your grocery list at first, and then reintroduce them after your symptoms have settled down to see if they affect you one way or the other.

Many grocery stores carry gluten-free breads and other products. When you're choosing restaurants, Indian, Mexican, and

Middle Eastern fare will have the most choices, and local celiac or gluten-free support groups will have restaurant recommendations for your area.

Depression

If you have an untreated depression, your memory may feel like it has been switched off. It's not just that you're in an emotional funk. Your brain can't seem to get in gear. But you will find that as depression lifts, either on its own or with medications, your memory will return to normal.

However, antidepressants are a mixed blessing, sometimes contributing to confusion and memory problems, as we saw above. I would suggest that you first explore nondrug treatments, particularly brief psychotherapy and exercise, and reserve medications for when these more natural methods do not do the job.

What Menopause Does to Your Brain

Many women do not feel like themselves as menopause approaches, and a common complaint is poor memory. If you were to have formal memory tests, however, you would likely find that your memory tests out fine. What is impaired at menopause is your concentration and your ability to learn, which are temporarily befuddled by the hormone shifts your body is going through. Luckily, these problems are temporary. As frustrating as they can be at the time, they will get better.

By the way, I strongly advise against taking hormone "replacement" therapy (HRT) in hopes of preventing memory problems or Alzheimer's disease. It does not prevent memory problems and may actually increase the risk of dementia. And HRT increases a woman's risk of stroke and breast cancer.

(continued)

If you are taking hormones for hot flashes, the treatment probably just postpones the hot flashes rather than eliminating them. The Women's Health Initiative was a large research study testing the effects of hormones, among other things. In May 2002, the hormone part of the study was abruptly cut short, due to emerging evidence of serious health risks. The 8,405 women who stopped their hormones were then surveyed. More than half of the women who had had hot flashes prior to beginning hormones found them recurring when the treatment was ended. So for most women, hormones are not a long-term solution to hot flashes.[4]

Alcohol or Drug Abuse

Not only does intoxication erase memories, but long-term drug or alcohol use destroys brain cells. If you are having more than one or two drinks a day, you're getting into the danger zone.

Thyroid Hormone—Too Little or Too Much

That humble little organ at the base of your neck affects so many things, from metabolism to memory. The memory problems caused by thyroid disease are not usually very severe, but they can occur. Blood tests will easily show whether your thyroid is making too little or too much thyroid hormone.

Symptoms of low thyroid (hypothyroidism) are often vague—fatigue, weakness, and weight gain. But if the condition continues, you could develop an enlarged thyroid, along with a wide variety of problems: dull facial expression, drooping eyelids, hoarse speech, dry skin, brittle hair, menstrual problems, slow heartbeat, constipation, depression, and anemia. Treatment with thyroid hormone is effective and is often helpful in borderline-low cases, too.

Overly high levels of thyroid hormone can affect memory,

too. Symptoms of hyperthyroidism include rapid heartbeat, pal- pitations, heat intolerance, weight loss, and menstrual irregulari- ties. You could also have an enlarged thyroid and appearance of unusually prominent eyes, among other problems. Treatment usually consists of medications, radioactive iodine, or surgery, followed by thyroid hormone replacement.

Thyroid problems sometimes improve on their own, without treatment. You will want to consult with your physician to see whether treatment is necessary.

Lack of Oxygen to the Brain

If the supply of oxygen to your brain is interrupted—even briefly—the results can be disastrous for the brain.

Perhaps the most dramatic situation is cardiac arrest. As the ambulance crew comes to your rescue and gets your heart beat- ing again, your family breathes a sign of relief. But while your heart was stopped, your brain cells were on their own. There was no oxygen reaching them, and the result could be persis- tent memory deficits.

Similarly, heart bypass surgery is often followed by cogni- tive problems. While the finger of blame had first pointed to the heart-lung machine (cardiopulmonary bypass), memory prob- lems occur even when the device is not used, suggesting that it may actually be due to some more fundamental problem in heart bypass surgery. The good news is that cognitive problems typically improve as the weeks go by.

Infections

Many kinds of infections can cause memory problems, so your doctor may think about several possibilities: Lyme disease, HIV, syphilis, and various kinds of encephalitis. The treatment is tar- geted to the specific organism.

Migraines

Many people with migraines feel that their headaches do real mischief to their memory and ability to focus. And indeed, researchers have found that people with migraines have trouble with verbal memory, reaction time, and even just paying attention, both during and after headache attacks.[5,6]

The good news is that treating the migraine gets your brain working again. Sumatriptan nasal spray (20 milligrams) rapidly restores cognitive function.[6]

As I mentioned above, you will want to see if diet changes can knock out your migraines. They often do. Common migraine triggers include dairy products, chocolate, eggs, citrus fruits, meat, wheat, nuts, tomatoes, onions, corn, apples, and bananas. Some of these foods (such as citrus fruits) are perfectly healthy for most people. But just as people who are allergic to, say, strawberries need to steer clear of them, the same is true of any food that is triggering headaches. With a simple elimination diet (described in my earlier book *Foods That Fight Pain*), it is easy to check which of these foods might be your culprit, and then you'll have power you did not have before.

Cancer Treatments

Chemotherapy often causes cognitive problems, in addition to its many other side effects. Researchers at the University of Toronto found that about half of women undergoing chemotherapy for breast cancer had moderate to severe problems with memory and language skills.[7] They also tested women who had finished their chemotherapy treatments more than a year earlier and found that about half had continuing cognitive problems that were at least moderate in severity.

Their memory problems were not psychological. That is, it

was not that depression or anxiety was interfering with their concentration. The problem was physical. Their brain cells simply were not working as well as they had before.

The fact is, chemotherapy is terribly toxic, which is exactly why doctors use it. They are trying to poison cancer cells. Unfortunately, some common chemotherapy drugs may be even more toxic to brain cells than to the cancer cells they are targeting.[8] As a result of these observations, many people are more and more cautious about chemotherapy.

Diabetes

Allow me to add diabetes to the list of memory threats. It is not that diabetes hurts your memory directly. Rather, people with diabetes are at heightened risk for Alzheimer's disease and stroke.

In 1988, Japanese researchers invited more than one thousand adults to have their blood sugar levels tested with a glucose tolerance test. They then followed them over the next fifteen years. Those whose tests showed them to be prediabetic—with fasting blood sugars that were above the normal range but not high enough for a diabetes diagnosis—were 35 percent more likely than other people to develop any sort of dementia. Those whose blood sugars were in the diabetic range were 74 percent more likely to develop dementia.[9]

Our research team has developed the most powerful dietary program ever devised for diabetes. Many people have used it to bring their blood sugar under better control and to reduce or even eliminate their medications. The regimen includes three simple steps: following a low-fat vegan diet, avoiding added oils, and favoring low-glycemic-index foods, as we will see in more detail in chapter 9.

Feeling Like Yourself Again

The conditions listed above are the most common problems affecting the brain. The list of potential problems also includes trauma, surgery, radiation, tumors, seizures, Parkinson's disease, Huntington's disease, and multiple sclerosis. In nonindustrialized countries, diets deficient in vitamin B_1 (thiamine) or vitamin B_3 (niacin) can also lead to serious memory problems, but these deficiencies are rare in developed countries, due to the widespread fortification of foods.

If you notice any change in your mental function, a check of the medicine cabinet and a good medical evaluation hopefully will identify the cause so that you can address it promptly.

PUTTING THE PLAN INTO ACTION

Now that you know about the brain-protecting effects of healthful foods, exercise, and attention to the effects of medicines and medical conditions, let me invite you to walk with me from the laboratory to the kitchen. It is time to put that knowledge to work.

In the next chapter, we'll trace out a brain-enhancing menu to give you optimal nutrition, along with a simple way to ease into it. We'll break the process into steps that are so simple that I have never seen anyone who couldn't follow them. Whether you like to cook or prefer to eat at restaurants—or even fast-food places—we've got you covered.

Next, we'll tackle food cravings—those annoying times when less-than-healthful foods just won't take no for an answer. I'll show you what these foods are doing inside your brain and what to do about it.

Finally, we'll arrive at a treasury of delightful recipes, devised by Christine Waltermyer and Jason Wyrick. Page through them, see which ones call out to you, and give them a try.

CHAPTER 9

A Brain-Enhancing Menu

Over many years, researchers have demonstrated the power of foods to help our hearts, trim our waistlines, tackle diabetes, ease chronic pain, and improve many other aspects of our lives. To this impressive list, we can now add protecting and enhancing our brains.

Luckily, you do not need one diet to bring you vitamins, a second to help you avoid "bad" fats, a third to limit iron exposure, a fourth for cholesterol control, and so on. One set of simple steps covers all these and more. This chapter puts it into action.

First, let me be clear about one thing: Nutrition is powerful. If you had imagined that a diet change might trim a few points off your cholesterol or help you lose a pound or two, it is time to think more boldly. Foods can change your life.

We have seen so many people who were hoping to just get their diabetes under a bit better control. They never suspected they might be able to reduce or even stop their medicines or that the disease could essentially disappear. We have seen people who have been beaten up by one failed weight loss regimen after another, only to learn that the failure was in those poorly designed diets, not in them, and that a new focus on truly healthful eating gave them more control than they had imagined possible.

The same is true with brain health. A few years ago, I would never have guessed that foods could have much effect on brain function or that they could change your odds for staying mentally clear into ripe old age. That is exactly what we are now aiming to do.

This prescription is not just healthful. It is also wonderfully enjoyable and diverse. As a child, I ate from a typical American diet, which, in retrospect, was very limited. We ate roast beef, baked potatoes, and corn, night after night after night. Sometimes a pork chop took the place of the beef or peas took the place of corn. But we knew nothing of the culinary brilliance of other lands and never explored the range of foods that nature makes available to us. As I began to move away from a meat-heavy diet to a plant-based menu, it felt as if the doors to truly delicious foods were finally opening up. As you page through the recipes in this book, you will see what I mean.

The Power of Food

Prior to 1990, most people thought modestly about nutrition. But that year, a page was turned. Dr. Dean Ornish, a young Harvard-training physician, showed that it is possible to actually *reverse* heart disease. Researchers had thought that artery disease was a one-way street. Narrowed vessels worsened over time, and surgery was the only way to reopen them. But, using a plant-based diet, along with other healthy lifestyle changes,

Dr. Ornish showed that, indeed, narrowed arteries can gradually reopen, reversing damage that had accumulated over decades.[1,2]

As revolutionary as Dr. Ornish's discovery was for the heart, it is potentially even more important for the brain. As you'll recall, about 20 percent of all the blood flowing from the heart passes up the carotid and vertebral arteries to the brain, carrying oxygen and nutrients in and carrying wastes out. Wide-open arteries are exactly what the brain needs.

Meanwhile, my research team tested the effect of a plant-based diet for obesity, diabetes, and cholesterol problems, all of which can harm the brain. It worked wonderfully. The participants slimmed down, their cholesterol levels dropped dramatically, their blood pressure improved, and many felt better than they had in years. Blood sugar control improved so much that some people with diabetes were able to stop their medications.[4]

Perhaps the biggest surprise was how our research participants felt about the diet change. After all, they were making what many would have thought was an enormous shift—throwing out the meat, dairy products, eggs, and oily foods. But they adapted quickly. They found delicious choices at restaurants and interesting new products at food stores, and came to see food in a whole new light. Their energy rebounded, and they felt great. They liked their new way of eating and were eager to keep it going permanently.

Even so, there can be occasional missteps along the way. In a study testing a plant-based diet for weight loss, we asked volunteers to set animal products aside and keep oils low, and we provided weekly group meetings to help everyone stay on track. In one of the first sessions, one of our participants announced, "Dr. Barnard, I've found a treat that I can have on your diet!"

"Uh-oh," I thought, running through the snack possibilities in my mind.

Opening her purse, she pulled out a big pack of red licorice. "Twizzlers!" she said. "Read the label!"

Twizzlers are pencil-shaped candy twists sold at convenience stores all over America. And it's true: If you look at the label, you'll find no animal ingredients and no added oil—they are just starchy, sugary, artificially colored junk food. And she made sure that the whole group knew that they could eat all the Twizzlers they wanted in Dr. Barnard's research study.

So my vegan, low-fat, Twizzler-fueled research participants set off on their path toward the unknown. Luckily, as the weeks went by, they lost weight. After fourteen weeks, the participants had lost an average of thirteen pounds.[3] And unlike the usual yo-yo effect seen with previous diets, weight loss became essentially a one-way street. Following them long-term, they were thinner after a year than when they began, and thinner at two years than at one year. Without counting calories, limiting portions, or even exercising, weight loss was easy and essentially permanent.

A Brain-Protecting Menu

A plant-based menu that is powerful for physical health is no less powerful for the brain. It allows you to skip "bad" fats, cholesterol, and excess metals that are linked to memory loss, while providing abundant vitamins your brain needs.

Let me lay out the guidelines for a menu that shields your brain, and then we will look at delicious breakfasts, lunches, and dinners that put these guidelines to work.

A Plant-Based Diet

It is best to avoid animal products *completely*. As you know by now, they contain saturated fat and cholesterol, increasing your cholesterol level and boosting your risk of Alzheimer's disease and stroke. While some people are tempted to include small amounts of meat, dairy products, or eggs here and there, those occasional animal products can easily stall your progress if you are aiming to lose weight, control cholesterol, and improve your brain health.

Some people use fish as a source of "good" fats, but fish also delivers cholesterol and a fair amount of saturated fat, as well as a surprising load of toxic pollutants in many species. As a group, fish eaters do not do nearly as well as people who focus on plant foods when it comes to weight, diabetes risk, and other health indicators.[5]

In 2009, the American Diabetes Association published a comparison of five different diet patterns in a study including 60,903 adults.[5] Some of them ate meat every day; others steered clear of it completely. Some had dairy products and eggs, or perhaps fish, while others avoided these foods. The researchers measured everyone's body mass index, which, as you will recall, is a measure of your weight, adjusted for your height (a healthy body mass index is between 18.5 and 25 kg/m^2).

The results were remarkable. People who ate meat daily averaged a body mass index of 28.8—well into the overweight range. Semivegetarians—that is, people who ate meat less than once a week—were slightly slimmer, with an average BMI of 27.3. People who ate no meat at all except for occasional fish were thinner than the first two groups but still in the overweight range. Those who left out all meats and fish but kept eating dairy products and eggs were thinner still. But the only group that was smack in the middle of the healthy weight range was the group of people who skipped animal products altogether. A plant-based (vegan) diet put their BMI at a healthy 23.6. The same gradient held for diabetes risk, too. In other words, the more people steer clear of animal-based foods, the healthier they are.

Planning Your Plate

To plan your brain-boosting menu, choose from each of the New Four Food Groups. These healthful foods are depicted in a simple graphic, called the Power Plate, which was developed by my organization, the Physicians Committee for Responsible Medicine.

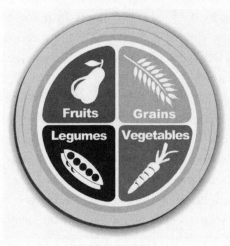

The Power Plate

Vegetables. As you plan your dinner, start with vegetables. They might be an afterthought for many people, but we will put them front and center. Have generous amounts—and why not two different ones, say, an orange vegetable, like carrots, and a green vegetable, such as broccoli or kale? And it's great to bring on fresh greens any time of day, whether in a salad, as a side dish, or perhaps added to a smoothie.

Vegetables are loaded with vitamins and give you minerals in the form your body can control. As you'll recall, plants have a special form of iron, called *nonheme* iron, which is more absorbable when your body needs more iron, and less absorb-

Vegetables That Cleanse the Blood

Certain vegetables have a special benefit. The group known as *cruciferous vegetables,* named for their cross-shaped flowers, includes broccoli, Brussels sprouts, cabbage, cauliflower, collards, kale, mustard and turnip greens, and watercress, as well as bok choy, kohlrabi, and rapini (broccoli rabe). They cause your liver to produce special enzymes, called phase 2 enzymes, that capture carcinogens and remove them from your bloodstream. The effect is quick, with enzymes increasing within twenty-four to forty-eight hours.

Sour + Bitter = Delicious. If broccoli, spinach, or other green vegetables are too bitter for your tastes, spritz them with lemon juice or apple cider vinegar. The combination of a sour topping with the slight bitter taste of vegetables creates a mellow, almost sweet taste you'll love.

able when you are already flush with iron (unlike the *heme* iron in meats, which tends to pass into your body whether you need it or not). That allows you to avoid the iron excesses that are implicated in Alzheimer's disease, among other health problems.

Whole grains. Next, add a grain, like rice, pasta, corn, or, if you prefer, a starchy root vegetable like sweet potatoes. These foods provide complex carbohydrates for energy, along with protein and fiber.

Legumes. Then add something from the legume group—beans, peas, and lentils—or any food made from beans, like tofu, tempeh, or hummus. They are loaded with protein and fiber, along with calcium and iron in their most healthful forms. They bring you traces of omega-3s, too.

How to Know If It's Organic

It is smart to favor organic produce, especially for those fruits and vegetables that are often dosed with pesticides. These include peaches, apples, bell peppers, celery, nectarines, strawberries, cherries, kale, lettuce, grapes, carrots, and pears.

On the other hand, the difference between organic and "conventional" is not as great for more disease-resistant crops that are less often chemically treated: onions, avocados, sweet corn, pineapple, mangoes, asparagus, sweet peas, kiwi, cabbage, eggplant, papaya, watermelon, broccoli, tomatoes, and sweet potatoes.

If you're having trouble figuring out whether produce is organic or not, just look for the little Price Look Up (PLU) sticker on the apple, orange, or whatever—the one cashiers use to check the price. If the number on the label starts with a 9, it's organic. If it starts with any other number, it is "conventionally" grown. If it starts with an 8, it is genetically modified.

Fruit. Finally, let's add some fresh fruit, either as dessert or as a between-meal snack: oranges, bananas, apples, tangerines, kiwis, mangoes, papayas—whatever strikes your fancy. How about some blueberries or strawberries to top your morning oatmeal? You might want to keep some extra fruit on hand—at

Finger Food

You may notice that uncut fruit tends to sit neglected on your counter, while finger-ready fruit rapidly disappears. If you pick up a cantaloupe or melon, cut it into chunks and leave a bowl of it in the refrigerator. You will find you're much more likely to take advantage of it.

home, in your office, or wherever you are—for anyone who might drop by.

Notice that so far, there is not a scrap of cholesterol or animal fat in your diet. The New Four Food Groups—vegetables, whole grains, legumes, and fruit—are a breath of fresh air for your brain and all the rest of you. They bring you powerful nutrition, and they skip what you don't need.

Needless to say, many recipes combine various food groups. Pasta is a grain that is topped with tomatoes, spinach, peppers, mushrooms, spices, or whatever else you are in the mood for. A burrito combines grains (a wheat tortilla) with beans (legumes), along with any vegetables you want to add, and maybe some fruit for dessert.

Take a look through the recipes in the back of this book and see which ones appeal to you.

Be Careful About Oils, Too

As you're taking advantage of these healthful foods, it also pays to keep fats to a minimum. That is obviously true for animal fats and the trans fats (partially hydrogenated oils) that often end up in snack foods. But I would encourage you to keep added oils to a minimum, too, using the oil-free methods described below.

This is not a zero-fat diet, however. There are traces of natural fats in vegetables, fruits, and beans, and they deliver the good (omega-3) fats your body needs. And there are more concentrated omega-3s in flaxseed, flax oil, and walnuts. But if your diet is loaded with grease—corn oil, sunflower oil, safflower oil, soybean oil, and so on—their load of omega-6 fats competes with omega-3s for the enzymes your body uses to lengthen them. That means your omega-3s have a hard time converting to the DHA your brain is looking for.

Don't get me wrong. Vegetable oils are nowhere near as unhealthful as animal fat. Researchers with the Chicago Health and Aging Project found that people who favored vegetable oils had a much lower risk of Alzheimer's disease compared with people favoring animal fats. Even so, most of us are inundated with oil we don't need, and it is a good idea to degrease your diet.

When fruits and vegetables are plucked from trees or from the earth, most have only traces of fat, and very healthful ones at that. There are a few exceptions in the plant kingdom: nuts, seeds, olives, avocados, and soy products have more substantial amounts of fat, so you'll want to be cautious. A small handful of nuts is about 1 ounce. That's a reasonable daily limit.

Simple Tips for Fat-Free Cooking

Sauté onions, garlic, mushrooms, and similar foods in vegetable broth or water instead of oil. Better yet, you can sauté in a dry pan. Try it and you'll see.

Steaming vegetables preserves their flavor without adding fat.

Steer clear of fried snacks. Potato chips, french fries, and other snack foods deliver a huge load of hidden fat. Baked versions are better.

Top your toast with jam instead of butter or margarine. Or if your toast started out as a really good bread, you won't need any topping at all.

Grocery stores now offer dozens of fat-free salad dressings. Or splash on some seasoned rice vinegar or other flavorful versions (such as balsamic or apple cider vinegar). A squirt of lemon juice goes great on salads and green vegetables.

If you are shopping for commercially prepared products such as frozen dinners, favor those with less than 3 fat grams per serving.

Go for the Vitamins

So we're using the New Four Food Groups and keeping oils low. And now, as you're filling your plate, you'll want to pay special attention to foods that provide brain-nourishing vitamins. Here are two easy tips that help you do that:

• Favor vegetables—especially green leafy vegetables, cooked or raw, along with beans and fruits. They deliver plenty of folate and vitamin B_6.

• Sprinkle a few nuts or seeds on your salad and you'll get vitamin E. Good choices are almonds, walnuts, hazelnuts, pine nuts, pecans, pistachios, sunflower seeds, sesame seeds, and ground flaxseed. About 1 ounce (one modest handful) per day will do it. Vitamin E is also in broccoli, spinach, sweet potatoes, and mangoes.

So it's easy to have a vitamin-rich menu. Focus on vegetables, fruits, and beans, and have a sprinkle of nuts and seeds here and there. You will also want to be sure to have a B_{12} supplement or B_{12}-fortified foods, as described below.

Veggies and Blood Thinners

People who are treated with a blood thinner called warfarin (sold under the brand name Coumadin) sometimes are told by their doctors to avoid vegetables. Here is what their doctors are thinking: Warfarin prevents blood clots by blocking vitamin K. But vegetables supply vitamin K, so some doctors worry that they will interfere with this anticlotting effect.

(continued)

If you take warfarin, speak with your doctor. The answer might not be to avoid vegetables but simply to keep the amount of vegetables you eat more or less steady from day to day. That way the blood tests your doctor uses to set your warfarin dose will stay fairly stable and your doctor will have an easy time setting the dose that is right for you.

Tackle Toxic Metals

Okay, you're taking advantage of vegetables, fruits, whole grains, and beans, keeping oils to a minimum, and emphasizing the vitamin-rich choices. And now one last thing: Look out for toxic metals. As we saw in chapter 2, we'll want to avoid getting too much iron, copper, and zinc, and there is no requirement for aluminum at all. You're already steering clear of most toxic metals by basing your menu on foods from plants. They give you the copper, iron, and zinc your body needs, without the excesses. And here are some additional steps you'll want to take.

First, throw open your medicine cabinet or wherever you keep your multiple vitamins. If they contain iron, copper, or zinc, as most do, make a note to pick up a healthier product next time you're at the store. All health food stores sell B complex—supplements that provide the folate, B_6, and B_{12} you need, among other B vitamins. Or you could just get a B_{12} supplement, as a healthful diet will bring you plenty of folate and B_6. There is no need to take supplemental iron, copper, zinc, or other minerals unless your doctor specifically recommends them for a medical condition.

Before you close the medicine cabinet, read the label on any antacids you might be using so as to avoid aluminum. There is no shortage of aluminum-free brands.

Check the labels on breakfast cereals. Many have added iron, zinc, or other metals.

In choosing cookware, skip pans where aluminum or iron is in direct contact with food. And avoid aluminum-containing baking powder, something that is easy to do at home but more challenging at a pancake house where the cooks may not be reading the fine print on food labels. Ditto for frozen pizzas, where aluminum is often used in the cheese topping, and in single-serve packets of coffee creamer or salt.

Bottled springwater is safer than tap water, unless your water supply is tested as free of aluminum or you are using a reverse osmosis purifier, which will effectively remove aluminum. Avoid aluminum cans (yes, that includes soda and beer cans) and be careful about tea, which tends to contain aluminum, too.

Here's the Payoff

If it sounds like a big step to skip animal products and added oils and to emphasize healthful foods, it's actually easier than you might imagine. Flip through the recipes in the back of this book and you'll see how delightful your meals can be.

The payoff is huge. You've boosted your nutrition to a whole new level, minimizing the chances you'll ever have to deal with serious memory loss as the years go by. At the same time, your new menu helps you trim your waistline, lower your cholesterol and blood pressure, and control diabetes, all at the same time!

And now let me offer two more steps for extra credit. It turns out that certain foods have a special cholesterol-lowering effect, which is good for your heart and your brain. In addition, certain carbohydrate-containing foods are better than others. Here are the details:

Special Cholesterol-Lowering Foods

By now you know that a plant-based diet lowers cholesterol easily and impressively—after all, you're skipping the animal fat and cholesterol. But some foods go further, providing a special cholesterol-lowering effect.

Oats. If you've heard television commercials promoting the ability of oats to lower cholesterol levels, well, it's true. Their *soluble fiber* does the trick. Oatmeal and oat-based cold cereals (such as Cheerios) can shave extra points off your cholesterol.

When it comes to oatmeal, skip the instant and "quick" varieties and have old-fashioned instead. It still cooks up in just a few minutes. Steel-cut oats are also fine. Cook oatmeal with water, not milk. If you like your oatmeal creamy, stir the oats into cold water and wait for a minute or two before bringing them to a boil. If you like it crunchier, boil the water first, then stir in the oats. Top with cinnamon, raisins, sliced bananas, strawberries, or whatever your tastes call for.

If you chose cold cereals, top them with soy milk, almond milk, rice milk, or other nondairy milk rather than cow's milk.

Beans. Not only are beans rich in protein, calcium, and healthful nonheme iron, they also have plenty of cholesterol-lowering soluble fiber. You don't need a huge serving. Four ounces is more than enough. People who eat beans regularly have cholesterol levels that are, on average, about 7 percent lower compared with their bean-neglecting friends.[6]

So have baked beans, black beans, hummus (made from chickpeas), split pea soup, lentil soup, or whatever other varieties you like. If beans cause a bit of gassiness, just have smaller servings and be sure they are cooked until very soft. Over time, this tends to sort itself out.

Barley. Barley is often used in soups and in breakfast cereals, and it lowers cholesterol, too, for exactly the same reason. Barley has plenty of soluble fiber. Add it to your own soup recipes, or mix it with rice. It tastes great and lowers your cholesterol as a bonus.

Soy. Soy milk, edamame, tofu, and tempeh were perfected in Asia, and have now found a huge audience in the West. Apart from the fact that they replace cholesterol-laden meats and dairy products, soy products seem to have a cholesterol-cutting effect of their own.[7]

Almonds and walnuts. People who eat almonds and walnuts regularly tend to have lower cholesterol levels compared with people who skip them.[8] As I mentioned above, I suggest limiting nuts to about 1 ounce per day and using them as an ingredient or topping rather than a snack.

Cholesterol-lowering margarines. Certain margarines block the absorption of cholesterol from the intestine. Benecol Light, for example, is made with plant *stanols* that come from pine trees, and it has a cholesterol-lowering effect. But like nuts, these products are fatty and should be used sparingly.

At the University of Toronto, Dr. David Jenkins put these foods to the test. He asked a group of patients to avoid animal products and to include foods like oats, beans, barley, soy products, almonds, walnuts, and special margarines in their routines. Their LDL ("bad") cholesterol dropped like a stone, falling nearly 30 percent in four weeks—essentially the same drop as is seen with cholesterol-lowering drugs.[9]

Choose Healthful Carbohydrates

This is not a low-carbohydrate diet, and for good reason. *Your brain runs on carbohydrates.* Just as your car runs on gasoline, your brain and all the rest of you needs *glucose,* the natural sugar that is released as starchy foods are digested.

The healthiest, slimmest, longest-lived people on Earth—and those who tend to keep their mental faculties lifelong—are those who include plenty of carbohydrate-rich grains, beans, noodles, fruits, and starchy vegetables in their routine.

If you have subscribed to the "carbohydrates-are-fattening" myth, the fact is that they have only 4 calories per gram, compared with 9 calories per gram for any kind of fat or oil. So why have carbs gotten a bad name? The reason is that we tend to combine them with grease. A cookie, a cake, or a pie does have some carbohydrates in the form of flour or sugar. But it is the stick of butter or cupful of shortening in a batch of cookies or a cake that really packs in the calories.

So carbohydrates are not fattening. Even so, the carbohydrate category is enormous, including everything from fruit, pasta, and breads to candy and sodas, and some carbs are better than others. Here are tips for choosing the best ones.

Natural and unprocessed. Brown rice has all the fiber nature could pack into it. But when the outer bran layer is removed to turn it into white rice, the fiber is mostly gone. Same with wheat when it is refined to produce white flour. Generally speaking, whole grains are better than those that have had their natural bran milled away.

Low glycemic index. Certain foods cause your blood sugar to rise more quickly, while others are gentler on your blood sugar. The glycemic index sorts out which are which. The glycemic index was invented in 1981 by Dr. David Jenkins—the same innovative scientist who showed how a portfolio of foods could slash cholesterol levels.

The glycemic index is calculated by feeding a given food to volunteers and then tracking whether their blood sugar rises steeply or gently. Foods that cause blood sugar to spike—that is, "high-GI" foods—can be a problem for people with diabetes. They can also cause triglycerides to rise, and some people feel that they accentuate cravings. In contrast, low-GI foods—foods that are gentle on your blood sugar—are easier on your system.

The GI champions are beans and green leafy vegetables. They have admirably low GI values, as do barley, bulgur, and parboiled rice.

Some foods are surprises. Even though fruits are sweet, most have a very low GI. And pasta has a low GI, too. Yes, even white spaghetti. The reason is that it is so compacted in the manufacturing process that it digests very gradually and its glucose molecules are slow to pass into your bloodstream.

There are just a few high-GI foods to look out for. Here they are, along with good replacements:

• **White and wheat breads.** They tend to increase blood sugar. Rye and pumpernickel breads have lower GI values and are better choices.

• **White baking potatoes.** Big white potatoes tend to spike blood sugar. In contrast, yams and sweet potatoes are gentler on your blood sugar.

• **Most cold cereals.** Puffed up, sugary cereals spell blood sugar problems. In contrast, bran cereal is easy on your blood sugar, as is oatmeal.

For many people, the glycemic index of foods is a secondary issue; that is, they can handle both high- and low-GI foods pretty well. However, if you have diabetes, weight problems, or high triglycerides, you'll do well to favor low-GI foods.

How Do I Get Started?

By now, you might be thinking that it sounds like a tall order to rethink your menu. After all, I'm suggesting you break some habits you've carried with you for a very long time. Let me show you a trick that we use in our research studies to help people adopt a new diet. It's easy. We just break the transition into two steps:

First, check out the possibilities. Don't change your diet yet. Take a week or so to see what you like. The idea is to find foods that fit the guidelines we talked about and that fit your tastes, too. I suggest taking a piece of paper and writing down four headings: breakfast, lunch, dinner, and snack. Under each heading, fill in foods that are free of animal products and are healthful overall—foods that you might like to try. Browse through the recipe section and see what calls to you.

Breakfast might be Blueberry Buckwheat Pancakes or Waffles topped with bananas or fresh blueberries and maple syrup. Or how about a bowl of old-fashioned oatmeal with sliced strawberries and crushed walnuts? Perhaps bran cereal with almond milk and banana chunks? If you're a sausage lover, skip the Jimmy Dean and make it Gimme Lean. Yes, that's the veggie sausage that has taken over a big corner of the market because it tastes just like sausage, without the oink or the cholesterol.

Take a minute, think what you might like for breakfast, and write it down.

For lunch, soups and salads are quick and tasty. How about Easy Quinoa Tabouli Salad, Easy Colorful Pasta Salad, or a big green salad, starting with whatever fresh greens your tastes call for, plus slices of tomato, cucumber, and fresh shiitake mushrooms (or any other variety)? Top with chickpeas and a sprinkling of slivered almonds. Then, how about Turkish Lentil Soup,

Mushroom Barley Stew, White Bean Chili, or Fresh Pea Soup? Perhaps a Baked Veggie Falafel sandwich, any of the many meatless versions of burgers and hot dogs, or perhaps a BLT (made with veggie bacon) with Dijon mustard on whole-grain bread.

If fast food is your thing, any submarine sandwich shop would be happy to make you a veggie sub with lettuce, tomato, spinach, olives, cucumbers, peppers, and a drizzle of red wine vinegar, and they'll even toast it for you. At the taco shop, skip the meat taco and have the bean burrito (hold the cheese).

At dinnertime, the sky's the limit. Salads and soups for starters if you like. Then how about Gnocchi with Basil and Sun-dried Tomatoes, Spaghetti with White Bean Marinara Sauce, Asian Stir-Fry with Apricot Teriyaki Sauce, Mexican Polenta Casserole, or Portobello Burgers? If it's pizza night, leave off the cheese and meat toppings and have all the veggie toppings, with extra sauce. And finish it off with Super Raspberry Protein Brownies, Baked Apples, Vanilla Berry Sorbet, or Chocolate Pudding.

The idea for now is just to see what you like. So jot down some ideas for breakfast, lunch, dinner, and snacks, and then take a week or so to test out recipes, convenience foods, or restaurant choices that fit our nutritional bill and satisfy your tastes.

A three-week test-drive. Once you know which foods you like, the next step is to take your new menu for a three-week test-drive. During this time, the idea is to follow the guidelines 100 percent—skipping the animal products and added oils, and really focusing on healthful foods. This is a twenty-one-day vacation from whatever less-than-perfect habits have clung to your pants leg all these years.

After three weeks, size up your progress. Chances are you will have shed unwanted weight, your cholesterol and blood pressure will be better, and your energy will be up, too.

You might also discover that your tastes are changing. You did not count on that, but it happens. The old, unhealthy foods start to seem—well, old and unhealthy. Your taste for grease is rapidly falling away. And you're on the path to better health.

Whether you can sense it or not, all the "side effects" of your menu change are good ones. The arteries in your heart are opening up, your cancer risk is plummeting, the likelihood you'll ever develop diabetes is falling (or if you have diabetes now, it is coming under better control). Weight control becomes easier than ever. And you're discovering new tastes that will soon become your best friends.

Quick Shopping Tips

Modern life is getting faster. More and more people have their breakfast in the car on the way to work and survive on fast food at lunchtime. "Home cooking" doesn't go much further than microwaving a pizza. We keep the same pace on our days off. People nowadays eat on the go practically nonstop.

Now, you are probably imagining that I will tell you to stop, take a breather, and live in the moment. But that is not my message. Life is not slowing down, and neither are you. And why should you? There is no reason you cannot enjoy a fast-paced life and eat healthfully at the same time. If you are spending hours at the store, let me offer a few tips to get you out the door quickly:

- **Stock up, and shop less frequently.** If you pick up larger quantities of healthful staple foods and keep them on hand, you can cut way down on your trips to the store. Rice, oats, and other grains keep well. Ditto for frozen vegetables, canned beans, pasta, and tomato sauce. Look for tofu in shelf-stable packaging (as opposed to water-packed tofu); unopened, it lasts for months. The same is true for soy milk, rice milk, and other dairy-free milk products.

- **Get in, get out.** If you have a shopping list in hand as you walk in the store, you'll be out the door faster and will be less susceptible to impulse purchases. You'll also save yourself a repeat trip for items you forgot to buy.
- **Let the store do the work for you.** Many stores sell varieties of premixed salad greens, along with frozen precut broccoli, cauliflower, beets, and so on, all of which will save you time in the kitchen. If you enjoy carrot juice, baby-cut carrots will save you the labor of scrubbing regular carrots.
- **Get groceries at the salad bar.** If you just need a few items, check out the salad bar. You'll have exactly what you need, with zero preparation time and no waste.
- **Let your mouse do your shopping.** In many cities, you can pick out your groceries online—even perishables, like fresh produce—and have them delivered to your door for a nominal charge. It's simple, and once you've submitted an order, you can save your preferences and modify future orders as you wish. Peapod (peapod.com) and Safeway (shop.safeway.com) are two common services, and you'll find others convenient to you.

What Supplements Should I Take?

Foods give you the nutrients your brain and body need. But there are a few supplements you should know about, too.

Vitamin B_{12}. As I mentioned in chapter 4, everyone should have supplemental B_{12} in their diets. This is not optional. The US government recommends it for everyone over age fifty, and I would recommend it for everyone, regardless of age.

Vitamin B_{12} is in many fortified cereals and fortified soy milk, and those sources are perfectly fine. For convenience, the easiest source is a multiple vitamin. Choose a brand that does *not* have added minerals. Drugstores and health food stores also sell supplements with just B_{12} alone or "B complex" (that is, a mixture of B vitamins), and they will do fine. Any brand you find in a store will have more than the 2.4 micrograms you need, and there is no toxicity from supplements with higher amounts.

Folate and vitamin B_6. If blood tests show that your homocysteine level is high, it may be sensible to add folate and B_6 to your regimen. As we saw in chapter 4, Oxford researchers used a combination of 800 micrograms of folate and 20 milligrams of vitamin B_6, along with 500 micrograms of vitamin B_{12} in people with high homocysteine levels. The vitamin combination reduced homocysteine and boosted their cognitive function. If you do not have a high homocysteine level, you'll get the folate and B_6 you need from foods alone.

Vitamin D. Although vitamin D's best-known function is to help you absorb calcium from the foods you eat, it also has an anticancer effect that is worth knowing about. The natural source is sunlight. Fifteen or twenty minutes of direct sunlight on your face and arms each day gives you all the vitamin D you need. But if you are indoors most of the time, you'll want to take a supplement. The US government recommends 600 IU per day for adults up to age seventy and 800 IU per day for people older than seventy.

Because of vitamin D's cancer-preventing effects, some authorities recommend daily doses as high as 2000 IU per day. This level of supplementation appears to be safe, but do not exceed that dose without a physician's directive.

DHA. As we saw in chapter 3, your body makes the DHA

your brain needs. However, some people hedge their bets with a DHA supplement. If that includes you, it is best to choose a vegan brand (as opposed to fish-derived brands) and to have 100 to 300 milligrams per day.[10]

Beyond Food

So you're babying your brain with healthful vegetables, fruits, legumes, and whole grains, and giving it the vitamins it needs. You're skipping animal products, added oils, and toxic metals, and your brain is thrilled. You are now miles ahead of most other people.

But while a healthful diet is Step One of our brain-protecting program—and it gives you enormous power—don't forget Steps Two and Three. Step Two is to exercise your brain and body. That means regular mental stimulation through reading, puzzles, and social interaction, or one of the specially designed online programs mentioned in chapter 5. These cognitive activities are enriching in every way, in addition to their ability to strengthen the connections in your brain.

And be sure to get your heart pumping, once your doctor gives you the okay. Begin slow—a ten-minute walk each day is fine for starters, and keep your pulse in the safety zone you calculated in chapter 6. Then, each week, increase your duration by five minutes until you are exercising for forty minutes at a stretch. Focus on your pulse, not on distance, and stop whenever you need to. And be sure to put exercise on your calendar if you have not done so already.

Step Three is to tackle physical threats—sleeplessness, medication side effects, and medical problems that can harm your brain.

When the clock strikes 10 p.m., turn out the light and go to sleep. You'll wake up refreshed, and you'll notice the benefits for memory, mood, and overall well-being. If sleep is a problem for you, carefully review the guidelines in chapter 7 to get you back on track.

If you are on medications that could affect your memory or cognition, check with your physician regularly to see if you really need them, paying special attention to those listed in chapter 8. Also be attentive to the medical conditions listed in that chapter. Your doctor will help you.

Now your menu is in good shape, you're putting your brain and body through their paces, and you're giving special attention to sleep and medical issues. You've done yourself a huge favor, and your brain and body will thank you.

But we're not quite done. In the next chapter, we'll tackle what, for many people, is the biggest issue of all—sticking with a healthful diet over the long run. We'll learn how we go astray and how to stay on track.

CHAPTER 10

Conquer Food Cravings

Have you ever been attracted to a food that you knew was not good for you? Did you ever dig into a greasy burger, a triple-cheese pizza, a candy bar, or double-chocolate cake, knowing that they could affect your weight or clog your arteries?

Of course. We've all been there. Even when we know that some foods are not doing our bodies any favors—maybe even *especially* when we know they are bad for us—we are like moths to a flame.

Why does that happen? It is perhaps the single most important question we could ask. Sometimes understanding the facts about what can destroy or protect the brain is not enough to motivate us to action, and we need more incentives to eat right.

The fact is, a war is going on inside your brain, and one small part of your brain is winning. Its weapon is *dopamine*. It can kill your resolve to stay healthy, and it may end up killing *you*. Let's take one last trip to England, where we'll spot the problem.

Just as the Beatles hit the peak of their popularity, the drug culture was exploding. In San Francisco, New York, London, and everywhere else, marijuana, hallucinogens, cocaine, and heroin were becoming widely available for the first time, and society was trying to sort out how to deal with them.

Musicians seemed especially vulnerable to the deadly effects of drugs and alcohol. Jimi Hendrix, Janis Joplin, Jim Morrison, and Rolling Stones guitarist Brian Jones were all part of the so-called 27 Club, named for their age at death. "We were smoking marijuana for breakfast," John Lennon said in a 1980 interview.[1] "We were well into marijuana and nobody could communicate with us, because we were just all glazed eyes, giggling all the time. In our own world." Cocaine, LSD, and alcohol all came along, too.

Now, a key part of a manager's job is to fend off drugs, alcohol, and any other threat to success, or at least to try to contain them as much as possible. After all, if the band stops showing up for gigs or cannot make it through a performance, the game is over.

But Epstein—the forward-thinking, exquisitely organized planner who always seemed to know the best path forward—did not stop the Beatles' drug use. He couldn't, because he was pulled into the world of drugs himself.

Perhaps it was inevitable. Drugs were everywhere in the music business at that time. Moreover, Epstein pushed himself to the absolute limit. Most people would have been satisfied to be managing the most successful musical group in history. But Epstein simultaneously took on another Liverpool group— Gerry and the Pacemakers—and guided them to stardom with "Ferry Cross the Mersey" and many other hits. He also managed Billy J. Kramer and the Dakotas and Cilla Black, merged with the management company that handled Cream, the Who, and the Bee Gees, launched a theater, and took on endless other projects. For a young man who had fallen into the music business by taking a job in his parents' furniture store's record department, success came dizzyingly fast. Drugs became a coping mechanism. Epstein fell into amphetamines, marijuana, and barbiturates, experimented with heroin, and sometimes drank more than was good for him.[2]

On August 27, 1967, Brian Epstein did not answer his phone. A knock on his apartment door elicited no response. His live-in assistant broke open his bedroom door and found his pulseless body lying on his bed. The medical examiner took blood samples, which revealed Carbrital, a barbiturate.

This was not a suicide. Barbiturates had been Epstein's way to turn off his brain and get to sleep, and over time it took more and more to shut out the day's events.

So 1967 did not bring us a picture of the sober manager who reined in the rowdy rock band and kept them on the straight and narrow. Epstein was drawn into the world of drugs and was ultimately destroyed by them.

Why Do You Think They Call It Dopamine?

If drugs are so deadly—if they can get you into trouble with the law, destroy your relationships, ruin your career, and maybe even kill you—why do people take them? The reason is dopamine.

Deep inside your brain, in what is called the *reward center*, dopamine waits in tiny round vesicles inside brain cells. Dopamine is a neurotransmitter. That is, it is a natural chemical that carries messages from one brain cell to another. It is actually waiting for you to find something to eat—some really good, tasty food. As soon as you do, dopamine bursts out from one brain cell and races across the gap to give the news to a neighboring cell. Other brain cells follow suit—one cell squirting dopamine at the next, all of which creates a little party in your brain and a feel-good sensation for you.

Your brain is not doing this just for fun. Your brain uses dopamine to make sure you remember the sights, sounds, and smells of this happy event, so that you'll come back and do the same tomorrow. After all, food keeps you alive. Dopamine resets your priorities to make sure that whatever else you might have had on your schedule—battling a neighboring clan, planting a garden, flying to the moon, or whatever—it will all come second to whatever got your dopamine flowing. Dopamine organizes your to-do list.

If this sounds odd, it is important to remember that for much of our time on Earth, food was not just sitting at the corner grocery store. You had to go out and find it, and you had to be able to separate what was nourishing from what was poisonous. And so the reward center has been part of the mammalian brain since long before the dawn of our species. Our biological cousins use it, too. At Gombe, on the shores of Tanzania's Lake Tanganyika, Jane Goodall observed chimpanzees digging into the succulent strychnos fruit. As the juice dripped down their chins, you could almost see the dopamine sparks in their brains.

Your reward center is also keen on sex. No, sex doesn't keep you alive, but it goes a long way toward keeping the species alive, so it has gotten favorable treatment as evolution shaped our brains.

So your reward center is looking for food and for a receptive mate, and when it finds them, out comes the dopamine. But this primitive system can be hijacked by drugs. A whiff of marijuana, a snort of cocaine, a shot of heroin, and, in fact, virtually all drugs of abuse trigger the release of dopamine. The same is true of a glass of wine, a cigarette, and a cup of coffee. Whatever else they do in your brain—calm you down, pick you up, create hallucinations, ruin your driving, or anything else—they also trigger dopamine. That's why people use them. The market for legal and illegal drugs depends on a flaw in the human brain: Its dopamine switch is easily manipulated.

Foods as Drugs

Drugs are *much* more potent at triggering dopamine compared with foods or sex, which is why addicts often lose interest in food, sex, and more or less everything else in favor of their drug of choice. But food manufacturers found that they could play that game, too. The dopamine release that you get from an apple, an orange, or a strychnos fruit is actually pretty modest. So, over time, the food industry has learned how to enhance it, making products that are less and less like food and more like drugs.

Exhibit A: sugar. Yes, an apple or an orange is pleasantly sweet, and it tastes very nice on a hot summer day. But why stop there? By extracting and purifying the juice from sugarcane or sugar beets, sugar companies get pure, concentrated *sucrose*—table sugar. And sugar is a hit. We bake it into cookies, pies, and cakes, and give it to children to show our "love."

In the brain, sugar stimulates the release of mild opiates— that is, natural compounds that are in the same chemical class as heroin and other narcotics but much weaker. You probably already know of some of the opiates the brain creates—the natural endorphins that cause the "runner's high" that marathoners experience. Sugar also stimulates the release of dopamine.

Exhibit B: chocolate. In prehistoric Central America, Aztecs turned cacao beans into a warm drink they called *chocolatl*. It was bitter, and neither they nor the early Spanish explorers saw much commercial potential in it. But in the mid-1800s, chocolate manufacturers discovered that by extracting and concentrating cocoa butter and then combining it with cocoa powder, sugar, vanilla, and other flavorings, chocolate becomes irresistible. Dopamine receptors light right up.

Exhibit C: cheese. Cows produce milk for one reason: to nourish their young. But about ten thousand years ago, some adventurous humans decided to taste cow's milk themselves. In your digestive tract, milk's *casein* protein breaks apart to release mild opiates, called *casomorphins*. They are not produced by your brain cells. They are actually in the milk protein that nature meant for the rapidly growing calf, and as you digest it, the opiates are released and absorbed into your bloodstream. In turn, these opiates trigger dopamine release.

Later on, someone figured out that coagulating milk and expressing out the water transforms it into cheese. And now we're on to something. Cheese has concentrated casein and so delivers a much larger casomorphin dose. It may smell like old socks and have more saturated fat, cholesterol, and sodium than a steak, but people flock to the cheese counter to get their hit of opiates and dopamine.

Exhibit D: meat. Humans do not have the long canine teeth that natural carnivores like cats and dogs use to kill and dismember prey. At least three and a half million years ago, our ancestors' canine teeth withered away to be no longer than their incisors. So while we were pretty handy with fruit, leaves, nuts, and anything else we could pick with our fingers and opposable thumbs, dismembering a mastodon was not really in the cards. Then, when the Stone Age brought us hatchets, arrowheads, axes, and knives, we finally were able to eat like carnivores. Never mind that we still have pre–Stone Age bodies that develop heart disease and colon cancer in response to meat eating. Meat, like sugar, chocolate, and cheese, has an opiate effect in the brain, which in turn triggers dopamine release. Researchers have shown that when people are given a drug that blocks opiate effects in the brain, they lose much of their interest in meat.[3]

So let's come back to the question that started us off: Why do we eat foods that we know are not good for us? Because they bathe our brains in dopamine. And dopamine won't take no for an answer. It glamorizes every last detail of whatever triggered it—the sweetness of sugar, the sizzle of a steak, and even the moldy smell of cheese.

Look at a wine connoisseur. At one point in his life, wine was not important to him. The first bitter taste might even have been a bit off-putting. But alcohol triggers dopamine, which embellishes every aspect of the drink that delivered it. He no longer speaks of how a wine smells; it now has a "bouquet." The color of the wine, its taste, its aftertaste, and the feel of the stem of the glass between his fingers—all engender glowing poetry, because they have been wildly oversold by dopamine.

Dopamine gets you into trouble. Up until now, good health, a long life, and a trim figure might have been high on your list of priorities, but chocolate, burgers, and cheese pizza elbow their way ahead of them. Have a candy bar—or two or three, your reward center tells you. Don't worry, just enjoy it, it insists.

So where is your Brian Epstein in all of this? Where's your internal manager who is supposed to talk you out of things you'll regret later? Unfortunately, dopamine got him, too. In fact, your cerebral cortex is recruited to help support the addiction. You'll find yourself coming up with increasingly far-fetched rationalizations for why you *ought* to set aside caution. "I can exercise those calories off," your now-corrupted brain tells you. "Everything in moderation," "My grandfather ate all the wrong things and lived to be ninety, so how bad can it be?" and so on. Your priorities have been reset, and your entire brain has been recruited to embrace the culture of dopamine.

There are certain times when you'll be especially susceptible to dopamine's siren call. When you are stressed, angry, lonely, or tired—when the world has treated you badly—you are not likely to look for solace in healthful foods. No one ever went to a convenience store at nine o'clock at night to buy cauliflower. That's when we turn to sugary cookies, chocolate bars, cheesy pizza, greasy burgers, or other junk food. We call them "comfort foods," because that is exactly the effect opiates and dopamine provide.

Some people are vulnerable for a different reason. Their genes conspire against them. During a research study on diabetes, I found that while some people changed their diets easily, others had a tougher time, and I wondered whether genes might explain this difference. It was already known that we all have a gene called DRD2—dopamine receptor D2—that is involved in building the receptors for dopamine. These receptors are like little docks on the outside of each cell, ready to receive the latest shipment of dopamine as it arrives. One variant of this gene causes you to have about one-third fewer dopamine receptors. And with fewer receptors, you do not get the same "feel-good" sensations other people get from dopamine. You would need an extra amount of dopamine just to feel normal. So you could end up being drawn to alcohol, smoking, drugs of abuse, and even risk-taking behavior, all of which give you an extra dose of the dopamine you are missing. About one in five people carries this genetic trait.

I took blood samples from each of our participants and sent

them to the University of California at Los Angeles, where Ernest Noble, MD, extracted their DNA. A short time later, Dr. Noble called me on the telephone. He had found that *nearly half of our diabetes patients had the gene variant that caused them to have too few dopamine receptors.*[4] That was far higher than the normal one-in-five prevalence of this genetic trait. Moreover, when we tracked how our patients did over time, those with the gene for too few dopamine receptors did not respond as well to a healthy diet—they did not improve as much—compared with people who had the normal number of receptors, presumably because they had more trouble with cravings and lapses.

I began to suspect that many people overeat in order to get dopamine stimulation. They are not aware of what is happening inside their brains, but they are drawn to food, especially unhealthful foods—more so than other people. They find it hard to break away. And when overeating gets into high gear, it leads to obesity, diabetes, and myriad other problems, including a higher risk of brain disorders.

If you are thinking you might like to be tested to see if your own food cravings could be due to a genetic trait, it is important to understand that *anyone* can fall victim to the addictive power of foods, no matter what genes you carry. Food manufacturers are doing everything they can to seduce your taste buds and keep you in a state of constant temptation with displays of food products in stores, gas stations, and airports and on television. They can easily overpower your inner manager, and they know it.

So am I saying that weight problems and diabetes are caused by dopamine? Yes, in part. And the same is true for heart disease, high blood pressure, and every other condition related to food, including Alzheimer's disease and stroke. In all of these conditions, the drive for dopamine draws you to the very foods that can hurt and kill you. It is dopamine that pushes you in front of the train.

Now, let's not be overly simplistic. Other genes play important roles in our disease risk, too, and even if you were on a perfect diet, you could still have health problems. Life is not fair. But eating healthfully goes a long way toward preventing health problems, and it is increasingly clear that there is a reason why unhealthful foods attract us. That reason lies deep inside our brain cells in tiny vesicles filled with dopamine.

Brian Epstein and Sigmund Freud

Is there a healthy way to get dopamine? Can we get a little bit of "feel good" without drugs, booze, or junk food? Well, I thought you'd never ask!

There actually are a couple of ways. First, you can break a sweat. Exercise releases mild opiates—endorphins—and also appears to trigger the release of dopamine. If you were to get up in the morning and have a half-hour run or a brisk walk, the natural feel-good sensation that comes from exercise would make you less likely to turn to unhealthful foods later in the day.

Second, there is a role for intimacy. If food is your preferred form of "comfort," it's time to have *real* comfort, which comes from developing friendships, engaging in conversations, intimacy, sexuality—any or all of the varieties of personal interaction.

But let's think beyond dopamine. Forty years before the Beatles and eight hundred miles away, Sigmund Freud wrote about the Beatles and Brian Epstein. He did not use their names, of course; they had not yet been born. But Freud described the unruly drives that well up from deep and primitive brain structures. For Freud, those scruffy, fun-loving, irresponsible, troublemaking desires were the *id*. And the manager—the more mature, forward-thinking part of ourselves—was the *ego*. The ego's job, like Epstein's, was not to frustrate the id. It was to help the id succeed. The ego makes plans, keeps you on schedule, and maintains the long view.

But the ego has limits, too, as Epstein illustrated so tragically. Freud wrote that there is a third brain function, called the *superego*. The superego is not there to manage your primitive drives. It looks beyond them, and helps you see the bigger picture around you. When you aspire to do good in the world, setting aside your own desires—that's the superego in action. And when you feel guilty about having let someone down, that's the superego, too. It is the part of you that thinks about others.

The ego—your manager—is not a particularly high-minded soul. The truth is, it just wants its percentage. That is, it helps you negotiate your world more effectively, and you'll both be better off. The superego is something else entirely. It looks at the needs of the world around us.

That broader view can save your life. It can provide the motivation you need to break away from unhealthy habits. Sir Paul McCartney described exactly this as he recalled looking out the window at his farm in Scotland. He was sitting with his wife Linda.

> We were eating roast lamb for Sunday lunch and it was the lambing season and there were all these beautiful little lambs gamboling around. Then we just looked at the lamb on our plate and looked at them outside again and thought "we're eating one of those little things that is gaily running around outside." It just struck us, and we said "Wait a minute maybe we don't want to do this." And that was it, that was the big turning point and we said we'd give up meat.[5]

This change of heart did not come from any sort of drive or ambition. This was not the id talking. Nor did it come from a manager prescribing a good career move or health advice. Paul and Linda began to consider the world around them. And then they realized how food choices affected their children, too.

> It was all brought into focus by our youngest daughter Stella coming home from school one day and saying how they'd been having this debate about eating meat and she said, "Mum, when we were talking about it I had a really clear conscience."

For most of human history, we did not need any dietary directives from our superego. Junk food simply was not available. We did not have an easy way to extract sugar from sugarcane or sugar beets, or to turn cacao beans into Snickers bars. Cheese hadn't been thought of, and meat eating, while not impossible, was arduous enough that steakhouses and chicken restaurants just were not a winning proposition. And when these products became available, it was a long time before they were inexpensive enough to be as ubiquitous as they are nowadays.

Today technology has removed those barriers. Junk food is cheap. We can have it anytime we want it. It calls to us from every corner, and that's where we run into trouble.

So I have two suggestions that are designed to help your ego and superego tackle that scruffy id of yours:

Set some rules. If you are having trouble resisting any unhealthful food, whether it's a greasy cheese sandwich, a chicken wing, or a sugary snack, you'll find it easier to set it aside completely than to tease yourself by having it occasionally. This is the opposite of what many people imagine. "Maybe I can just have it now and then," we say to ourselves. "A little bit won't hurt." And in theory, that's true. The problem is that each dose of a problem food triggers another dopamine blast that reinforces the desire for it. Each bite makes it harder to say no next time. By setting it aside—even for just a couple of weeks—we're able to forget about it a bit once we get over that initial craving hump.

If that sounds like tough love, it's exactly the lesson that smokers learned a long time ago. Quitting is not easy, but it is *much* easier than teasing yourself with an occasional cigarette. "Moderation"—for both cigarettes and junk food—is simply a way of stoking a fire rather than letting it go out.

Look to other motivators. Many people break the meat habit, not for themselves, but because they view factory farming and animal transport and slaughter as something they want no part of. Today Americans eat *more than one million animals per hour.* Even in my grandfather's day, it was not a remotely kind process, and today it is all the more miserable for all concerned.

Others are moved by reports of the environmental damage that modern factory-style farms engender. From the pesticides used to grow feed crops and the fecal output of chickens, hogs, and cattle that contaminate waterways, to the greenhouse gases emitted by the 100 million or so cattle grazing on American farms, raising livestock is no treat for Earth. These facts are motivating more and more people to change their diets.

One of the most common reasons people decide to take better care of themselves is that their spouses or children depend on them. Not only do we not want to burden our families if we become ill, we want to be there to help them through whatever problems they may encounter. We cannot afford to take risks with our own health that could mean abandoning them. And the more we model healthful habits, the more we help them to do the same.

Whatever your motivation for rethinking the contents of your plate, you will get a huge reward in the form of better health. And that will help you put dopamine in its place.

Go for It!

Now you know the secrets for keeping your brain and physical being well for a long and productive life. There are many recipes to sample, new tastes and new restaurants to try, and many things to explore.

I wish you the very best of luck, and I hope you will share what you've found with others.

CHAPTER 11

Menus and Recipes

The recipes that follow are the most delicious possible way to give your body and brain the nutrition they need. They are loaded with healthful vitamins and, at the same time, free of animal products, trans fats, and the overdose of toxic metals that are part of so many people's diets. They are also quick to prepare, using familiar ingredients, and each one comes with a nutrient analysis so you can see exactly what you're getting.

These recipes were developed by two inspired chefs with whom I have had the pleasure of working for years.

Christine Waltermyer is the founder and director of the Natural Kitchen Cooking School, where she provides chef's training programs, personal chef services, and in-home cooking classes in New York City and Princeton, New Jersey. She is a masterful chef with a particular gift for making healthful foods really appealing to people who may not have thought much about health before. She is a featured chef in PCRM's VIP Kickstart program offered to PBS supporters.

Jason Wyrick is the executive chef and publisher of the magazine *The Vegan Culinary Experience*. He has catered for companies including Google, the Frank Lloyd Wright Foundation, and many others, and has been a guest instructor in Le Cordon Bleu program at Scottsdale Culinary Institute. Jason has an amazing knack for flavor, combining natural ingredients with just the right spices to seduce the taste buds, and he makes cooking easy and quick for people with little time or cooking experience. Jason supplied the recipes for my previous book, *21-Day Weight Loss Kickstart*.

A Week's Worth of Menus

Day 1

Breakfast:

Blueberry Buckwheat Pancakes
  (page 195)
Veggie sausage
Fresh sliced cantaloupe

Lunch:

Garden salad with sliced
  tomatoes
Baked Veggie Falafel (page 219)
Pita bread

Dinner:

Red Lentil Soup in a Flash
  (page 202)
Brown Rice Salad (page 215)
Steamed spinach with lemon
  wedges
Fruit Pop (page 253)

Day 2

Breakfast:	*Dinner:*
Waffles with Maple "Bacon" (pages 195–96)	Spinach salad with slivered almonds
Lunch:	Tacos with Potatoes, Swiss Chard, and Pinto Beans (pages 223–24)
Easy Colorful Pasta Salad over mixed greens (pages 213–14)	Mashed sweet potato

Day 3

Breakfast:	*Dinner:*
Baked Oatmeal (page 197) with raisins	White Bean Chili with Red Rice (pages 206–7, 236–37)
Veggie bacon	Steamed spinach
Lunch:	Banana Ice Cream (page 248)
Tuscan Wrap (pages 220–21)	

Day 4

Breakfast:	*Dinner:*
Breakfast Wrap (pages 197–98)	Creamy Pumpkin Bisque (pages 203–4)
Fresh strawberries	That Delish Potato Dish (pages 239–40)
Lunch:	Steamed broccoli
Green salad	Chocolate Pudding (pages 255–56)
English Muffin Pizza (page 226)	

Day 5

Breakfast:	*Dinner:*
Polenta Breakfast Bar (pages 198–99)	Rainbow Salad with Strawberry Dressing (pages 212, 217)
Lunch:	Baked Ziti (page 229)
Easy Quinoa Tabouli Salad (page 213)	Warm Apple Cherry Compote (page 251)
Portobello Burger (page 220)	

Day 6

Breakfast:

Oyster Mushroom Frittata
   (pages 199–200)
Whole-grain toast

Lunch:

Mixed Greens and Spicy Roasted
   Tempeh (page 211)
Crusty bread

Dinner:

Curried Apple Daal Stew
   (page 209)
Toasted Brown Rice (page 236)
Steamed asparagus
Chocolate Pudding (pages
   255–56)

Day 7

Breakfast:

Smoothie Parfait (page 201)
Sliced banana

Lunch:

Creamy Pumpkin Bisque
   (pages 203–4)
Garbanzo Bean Sandwich
   (page 218)

Dinner:

Stuffed Peppers with Squash,
   Black Beans, and Rice
   (pages 234–35)
Moroccan Mint Couscous
   (page 239)
Super Raspberry Protein
   Brownie (page 254)

Breakfast

Blueberry Buckwheat Pancakes

Serves 2 to 4

These whole-grain pancakes drizzled with pure maple syrup make for a delicious and hearty breakfast. Blueberries add a delicious and healthful touch.

½ cup buckwheat flour
½ cup whole-wheat pastry flour
2 teaspoons flaxseed meal
1 teaspoon aluminum-free baking powder
Pinch of sea salt
1 cup rice milk
1 cup fresh blueberries
1–2 teaspoons safflower oil, to brush the skillet
Warmed maple syrup, for drizzling

In a medium bowl, combine the buckwheat flour, whole-wheat pastry flour, flaxseed meal, baking powder, and salt. Whisk briefly to blend. Slowly stir in the rice milk and stir just until the lumps disappear. Gently fold in the blueberries.

Heat a griddle or skillet over medium heat, then lightly brush with a little of the safflower oil. Add enough batter to form a 4-inch pancake and cook until the edges look dry and bubbly, about 2 to 3 minutes. Gently flip the pancake and cook on the other side until golden, about 2 to 3 minutes. Serve hot, with warmed maple syrup.

Per pancake: 82 calories, 2 g protein, 16 g carbohydrate, 3 g sugar, 1 g total fat, 13% calories from fat, 2 g fiber, 112 mg sodium

—CW

Waffles

Serves 4 (makes 4 waffles)

The aroma of cooking waffles will perfume your whole house.

1 banana
1 cup whole-wheat pastry flour

¼ teaspoon baking soda
½ teaspoon sea salt
2 servings Ener-G Egg Replacer with half the liquid called for on
   the package
1¼ cups almond milk or soy milk
1 teaspoon fresh lemon juice
Nonstick cooking spray

Freeze then thaw a banana and peel it. Mash the banana.

Preheat a waffle iron.

In a medium bowl, combine the flour, baking soda, and salt.

In another medium bowl, whip together the Ener-G Egg Replacer mixture and add the mashed banana, almond or soy milk, and lemon juice. Add the wet ingredients to the dry ingredients and combine them thoroughly.

Give the waffle iron a quick spray of nonstick cooking spray. Add some of the batter to your waffle iron (the amount depends on the size of your iron, but make sure the iron is covered with a thin layer of batter) and cook until golden brown, about 5 minutes. Gently peel the waffle out of the iron with a thin blade and repeat making waffles with the rest of the batter.

Per waffle: 143 calories, 4 g protein, 31 g carbohydrate, 2 g sugar, 0.3 g total fat, 2% calories from fat, 4 g fiber, 337 mg sodium

Here are three ways to add a bit of zing to waffles. When using ingredients like berries or nuts, stir them into the batter after the liquid and dry ingredients are combined.

Smoked Almond and Apple: Add ½ green apple, diced, and
   2 tablespoons chopped smoked almonds to the batter.

Maple "Bacon": Add 2 strips tempeh "bacon," diced, and
   2 teaspoons maple syrup to the batter.

Southwestern: Add 2 tablespoons diced roasted green chiles or
   rehydrated and diced ancho chiles to the batter.

—JW

Baked Oatmeal

Serves 4 to 6

This nourishing breakfast will start your day off right!

    2 cups rolled oats
    1 tablespoon flaxseed meal
    1 teaspoon ground cinnamon, plus more for serving
    Pinch of sea salt
    1½ teaspoons aluminum-free baking powder
    2¼ cups rice milk
    1 teaspoon pure vanilla extract
    ½ cup chopped dried apricots or raisins
    ½ cup fresh blueberries
    Rice milk, for serving
    Optional: 2 tablespoons maple syrup

Preheat the oven to 350°F and lightly oil an 8 x 8-inch baking pan.

In a large bowl, combine all the ingredients and stir until well combined. Pour into the prepared baking pan and bake uncovered for 30 minutes. Cool slightly, then cut into 8 squares. Serve warm, topped with a little rice milk and extra cinnamon.

Per serving (¼ of recipe): 285 calories, 7 g protein, 54 g carbohydrate, 17 g sugar, 5 g total fat, 15% calories from fat, 7 g fiber, 325 mg sodium

—CW

Breakfast Wraps

Serves 4

Looking for a healthy breakfast on the go? This wrap is easy to make and high in protein.

    1 14-ounce package firm tofu, drained
    2 cloves garlic, minced
    ½ cup diced onion
    1 teaspoon sea salt, or to taste
    ¼ teaspoon ground turmeric
    Freshly ground black pepper

4 whole-grain tortillas
½ cup prepared salsa

Place the tofu in a colander that fits inside a bowl. Put a small plate on top of the tofu. Add heavy weight, such as a few stacked bowls, on top to press the water from the tofu. Let the tofu sit for 10 minutes. Drain the tofu and crumble it into a separate bowl.

Heat a few tablespoons of water in a medium skillet over medium heat. Add the garlic, onion, and a few pinches of the sea salt. Cook for 5 minutes, until the onion is tender. Place the drained and crumbled tofu on top of the garlic and onion mixture. Sprinkle with the turmeric, the remaining sea salt, and pepper to taste. Cover the pan and cook for 3 minutes.

Place one-quarter of the tofu mixture in the middle of a tortilla. Add one-quarter of the salsa and wrap the tortilla tightly around the filling, securing it with a sheet of parchment paper if needed. Repeat with the remaining tortillas and filling.

Per serving (1 wrap): 201 calories, 15 g protein, 24 g carbohydrate, 2 g sugar, 7 g total fat, 29% calories from fat, 5 g fiber, 984 mg sodium

—CW

Polenta Breakfast Bars
Serves 4 to 6

These bars are easy to make in large batches and they store well and travel well, ideal for pulling out of the refrigerator as you run out the door!

2 cups water
1 cup yellow corn grits
1 tablespoon molasses
¼ cup agave nectar
Pinch of sea salt
1 teaspoon ground cinnamon
1 cup chopped walnuts
½ cup golden raisins
½ cup dried cranberries
Nonstick cooking spray

Boil 2 cups water. Reduce heat to medium-low, add the corn grits, and simmer for 5 minutes. Remove from heat and immediately add in the molasses, agave, and salt. Stir to combine. Stir in the cinnamon, walnuts, raisins, and cranberries.

Coat an 8½ x 4½ x 3-inch glass or metal dish with nonstick cooking spray (or use a high-quality nonstick pan). Transfer the mixture to the dish, cover, and refrigerate for at least 2 hours but preferably 6 hours or overnight. Either remove the entire hardened polenta cake from the dish and then slice it into bars, or slice it into 4 bars directly in the dish (but not if it's metal), and transfer to a plate to serve.

Per serving (¼ of recipe): 318 calories, 4 g protein, 66 g carbohydrate, 28 g sugar, 4 g total fat, 13% calories from fat, 5 g fiber, 6 mg sodium

—Recipe by Madelyn Pryor

Oyster Mushroom Frittata

Serves 2

A frittata is an Italian-style omelet. It is typically prepared on the stovetop and then transferred to the oven, or simply baked in the oven, creating a slightly crisped texture.

12 ounces extra-firm tofu
½ teaspoon ground turmeric
½ teaspoon sea salt
2 small red potatoes, diced
2 cloves garlic, minced
1 bunch spinach, chopped
6 green onions, sliced
Nonstick cooking spray
1 cup chopped oyster mushrooms

Preheat the oven to 375°F.

Put the tofu in a blender and add the turmeric and ¼ teaspoon of the salt. Blend until smooth.

Cook the potatoes in a sauté pan over medium heat with a very thin layer of water until they are only slightly softened, about

5 minutes. Add the garlic, spinach, and green onions and cook until the spinach has wilted, about 3 minutes.

Add the mixture to the blended tofu and divide the mixture between a pair of 4- to 6-inch ramekins or an 8-inch ovenproof skillet. Cover with foil and bake for 25 minutes.

While the frittata is in the oven, toss the mushrooms with the remaining ¼ teaspoon salt. Coat a sauté pan with cooking spray (or use a nonstick pan) and heat over high heat; add the mushrooms and sear them until they turn brown and slightly crisp, 4 to 5 minutes. Once the frittata comes out of the oven, top it with the oyster mushrooms and serve.

Per serving (½ of recipe): 173 calories, 12 g protein, 22 g carbohydrate, 2 g sugar, 5 g total fat, 28% calories from fat, 3 g fiber, 167 mg sodium

—JW

Breakfast Smoothie

Serves 2 (makes about 3 cups)

1 very ripe banana (with plenty of brown speckles)
2 cups frozen fruit (such as berries, mangoes, strawberries, banana, orange, and pineapple)
1 cup nondairy milk (almond milk or soy milk)

Combine all the ingredients in a blender. Start your blender on the lowest setting and slowly crank it up as the smoothie starts to puree. If you start with your blender at high, you'll end up with smoothie splattered all over the top of your blender and probably will have to stop your blender several times to get the smoothie ingredients to rest back on the blades. Once you're up to optimal speed, blend for about 2 minutes to get everything smooth.

Per 1½-cup serving: 190 calories, 2 g protein, 46 g carbohydrate, 35 g sugar, 2 g total fat, 9% calories from fat, 5 g fiber, 79 mg sodium

—JW

Smoothie Parfait

Serves 1

Adding toasted oats or granola to a smoothie means you can have your crunch and eat it, too.

¾ cup Breakfast Smoothie (page 200)
¼ cup toasted dried oats or granola
Fresh berries or a sprig of mint, for topping

Layer ¼ cup of the smoothie in the bottom of a glass. Add a 2-tablespoon layer of oats next, followed by another ¼ cup of smoothie, then the last 2 tablespoons oats, and finish it off with the last ¼ cup of smoothie. Top with fresh berries or a sprig of mint.

Per serving (using toasted oats): 303 calories, 104 g protein, 62 g carbohydrate, 36 g sugar, 2 g total fat, 7% calories from fat, 9 g fiber, 66 mg sodium

—JW

Soups and Stews

Red Lentil Soup in a Flash
Serves 6

Lentils are naturally quick to cook, and this clever recipe turns them into a delicious, nourishing soup you're sure to love.

½ cup diced onion
½ teaspoon minced garlic
1 teaspoon dried thyme
1 cup diced celery
1 cup diced carrot
2 cups red lentils, rinsed
1 bay leaf
7 cups low-sodium vegetable broth or water, plus more if needed
2 teaspoons balsamic vinegar
Freshly ground black pepper
2 teaspoons minced fresh parsley, for garnish

Heat 2 tablespoons water in a large saucepan over medium heat. Add the onion, garlic, and thyme and cook, stirring, for 5 minutes, or until the onion is soft and translucent. Add the celery and carrot and cook, stirring, for another 5 minutes. Add the lentils, bay leaf, and vegetable broth, increase the heat to medium-high, and bring to a boil. Decrease the heat to low, cover, and simmer for 20 minutes, or until the vegetables are tender. Add more broth as needed to achieve desired consistency.

Add the vinegar and pepper to taste. Cover and simmer for 5 minutes. Spoon into bowls and serve immediately, garnished with the parsley.

Note: As a time-saver, use your favorite vegetable chopping kitchen tool to cut up everything.

Per serving (⅙ of recipe): 236 calories, 16 g protein, 43 g carbohydrate, 6 g sugar, 0.8 g total fat, 3% calories from fat, 11 g fiber, 196 mg sodium

—*CW*

Mushroom Barley Stew

Serves 2

Barley has a nutty taste and makes for a filling stew. Because it tends to mute the flavors of other ingredients, this recipe is intentionally bold with spices.

½ yellow onion, diced

5 cremini mushrooms, sliced

2 cloves garlic, minced

2 cups water or low-sodium vegetable broth

1 teaspoon fresh thyme leaves

1 teaspoon paprika

½ teaspoon freshly ground black pepper

¾ cup barley (hulled or unhulled)

¼ teaspoon sea salt

Optional: 1½ cups baby spinach leaves or chopped kale

Place a medium saucepan over medium-high heat; add the onion and cook for about 10 minutes, until heavily browned. Add the mushrooms and cook for 3 minutes. Add the garlic and cook for 1 more minute. Stir in the vegetable broth and add the thyme, paprika, and pepper. Once the soup comes back to a boil (which will happen quickly), add the barley. Return the soup to a boil, cover the pan, reduce the heat to low, and cook for about 25 minutes. Remove from the heat and stir in the salt. If you are using the greens, add them when you add the salt and let them soften in the soup for about 3 minutes before serving.

Per serving (½ of recipe): 308 calories, 9.6 g protein, 68 g carbohydrate, 3 g sugar, 1 g total fat, 3% calories from fat, 14 g fiber, 270 mg sodium

—JW

Creamy Pumpkin Bisque

Serves 4

Nothing satisfies like a nice creamy soup. And this recipe can be adapted using cooked carrots, cauliflower, corn, potatoes, or any of your favorite vegetables.

1 cup diced onion

½ teaspoon minced garlic

4 cups low-sodium vegetable broth, nondairy milk, or apple cider

4 cups cooked or canned pumpkin puree

¼ teaspoon ground nutmeg

Sea salt and freshly ground black pepper

4 sprigs fresh parsley

Heat 2 tablespoons water in a medium saucepan over medium heat. Add the onion and garlic and cook, stirring, for 5 minutes, or until the onions are soft and translucent. Add the vegetable broth, then slowly add the pumpkin puree and nutmeg, using a whisk to blend, then use an immersion blender to blend until smooth. Add a little more broth if the soup is too thick. Season with salt and pepper to taste.

Decrease the heat to low, cover, and simmer for 10 minutes. Adjust the seasonings to taste. Serve hot, garnishing each bowl with a sprig of parsley.

Per serving (¼ of recipe, using vegetable broth): 77 calories, 2 g protein, 19 g carbohydrate, 13 g sugar, 0.3 g total fat, 3% calories from fat, 3 g fiber, 291 mg sodium

—CW

Potato Leek Soup

Serves 4

This rich-tasting soup is surprisingly low in fat, so go ahead and enjoy a steaming bowl.

4 leeks, white and light green parts, split lengthwise, washed, and sliced

1 teaspoon dried thyme

1½ pounds potatoes, peeled and diced

4 to 5 cups low-sodium vegetable broth

Sea salt and freshly ground black pepper

1 tablespoon minced fresh parsley, for garnish

In a large saucepan, heat 2 tablespoons water over medium-low heat. Add the leeks and thyme and cook, stirring, for 10 minutes. Add the potatoes and 4 cups of vegetable broth, raise the heat to medium-high, and bring to a gentle boil. Reduce the heat to low, cover, and simmer for 30 minutes. Remove from the heat and, using an immersion blender, puree at least half or all of the soup, depending on how smooth you like it. Add a little more broth if the soup is too thick. Season with salt and pepper to taste. Serve hot, garnished with the parsley.

Per serving (¼ of recipe): 183 calories, 4 g protein, 43 g carbohydrate, 7 g sugar, 0.4 g total fat, 2% calories from fat, 5 g fiber, 307 mg sodium

—CW

Creamed Corn Soup

Serves 4

Mmm…who doesn't love a bowl of piping hot soup? This one is sure to satisfy.

    2 cups diced onion
    4 cups corn kernels
    3 cups rice milk
    3 cups low-sodium vegetable broth
    1 cup diced zucchini
    ½ cup seeded and diced tomato
    Sea salt and freshly ground black pepper

In a large saucepan, heat 2 tablespoons water over medium-high heat. Add the onion and cook, stirring, for 5 minutes. Add the corn kernels and cook, stirring, for another 5 minutes. Slowly add the rice milk and vegetable broth, increase the heat to medium-high, and bring to a boil. Reduce the heat to low, cover, and simmer for 10 minutes. Remove from the heat and, using an immersion blender, blend until smooth. Increase the heat to medium-high and return the soup to a simmer; add the zucchini and tomato, reduce the heat to medium, and cook for 10 minutes, or until the zucchini is soft. Season with salt and pepper to taste.

Per serving (¼ of recipe): 263 calories, 7 g protein, 58 g carbohydrate, 20 g sugar, 3 g total fat, 10% calories from fat, 5 g fiber, 933 mg sodium

—CW

Fresh Pea Soup

Serves 4

Peas are high in protein and fiber and low in fat and calories. In this soup they provide a delicious, hearty taste.

1 cup diced onion

2 cloves garlic, minced

2½ cups low-sodium vegetable broth

2½ cups rice milk

4 cups fresh or frozen green peas

Sea salt and freshly ground black pepper

Fresh parsley sprigs, for garnish

In a large saucepan, heat 2 tablespoons water over medium-high heat. Add the onion and garlic and cook, stirring, for 5 minutes. Add the vegetable broth and rice milk, increase the heat to medium-high, and bring to a boil. Add the peas and cook for 5 minutes. Turn off the heat and, using an immersion blender, blend until smooth. Season with salt and pepper to taste. Serve hot, garnished with fresh parsley sprigs.

Per serving (¼ of recipe): 217 calories, 9 g protein, 41 g carbohydrate, 19 g sugar, 2 g total fat, 8% calories from fat, 8 g fiber, 803 mg sodium

—CW

White Bean Chili

Serves 4

Beans are nature's super food! They are rich in protein and fiber and help lower cholesterol. And they transform into this delicious chili.

2 cloves garlic, minced

1 cup diced onion

1 cup chopped celery

1 cup diced sweet potato

4 cups canned low-sodium white beans of your choice, drained and rinsed

2 teaspoons chili powder

1 teaspoon paprika
¼ teaspoon Tabasco sauce, or to taste
3 to 4 cups low-sodium vegetable broth
Freshly ground black pepper

Heat 2 tablespoons water in a large saucepan over medium heat.
Add the garlic and onion and cook, stirring, for 5 minutes, or until
the onion is translucent. Add the celery and sweet potato and
cook, stirring, for 5 minutes. Add the beans, chili powder, paprika,
and Tabasco sauce, followed by 3 to 4 cups of vegetable broth,
depending upon desired consistency. Increase the heat to medium-
high and bring to a boil. Cover, reduce the heat to low, and simmer
for 30 minutes. Season with pepper to taste.

Per serving (¼ of recipe): 308 calories, 19 g protein, 59 g
carbohydrate, 7 g sugar, 1 g total fat, 3% calories from fat, 14 g fiber,
166 mg sodium

—CW

Turkish Lentil Soup (Mercimek Corbasi)
Serves 3

Shredding the onion and carrot allows them to disappear into this
classic Turkish soup, giving the broth a full-bodied flavor with the
smooth texture of soft red lentils.

1 onion, shredded or diced
1 carrot, shredded or diced
2 cloves garlic, minced
4 cups water or low-sodium vegetable broth
3 tablespoons low-sodium tomato paste
2 tablespoons diced roasted red pepper
½ teaspoon crushed red pepper
1 cup red lentils
Optional: 1 tablespoon chopped fresh mint

Heat a large saucepan over medium heat. Add the onion and carrot
and cook until the onion is lightly browned, about 5 minutes. Add the
garlic and cook for another minute. Add the water or broth, tomato
paste, roasted red pepper, and crushed red pepper, stirring everything

together until it is thoroughly combined. Once the liquid is simmering, add the lentils. Bring to a boil, cover the pot, and reduce the heat to low. Cook for 25 minutes, then remove from the heat and serve, garnished with the mint, if desired.

Per serving (⅓ of recipe; prepared with water): 440 calories, 27 g protein, 81 g carbohydrate, 10 g sugar, 1 g total fat, 3% calories from fat, 32 g fiber, 237 mg sodium

—JW

Enchilada Bean Soup
Serves 2

In this soul-satisfying, thick soup, red beans are pureed with enchilada sauce and garlic and thickened with corn tortillas. It even makes a great dip or burrito filling!

¼ cup mild chili powder
2 tablespoons whole-wheat pastry flour or masa harina
2 teaspoons ground cumin
2 cups canned low-sodium red beans, with liquid
2 cloves garlic
2 corn tortillas, torn into pieces
Optional: 1 or 2 chipotles in adobo sauce; 1 tablespoon
   chopped fresh oregano

Combine the chili powder, flour, and cumin in a medium saucepan. Place over medium heat and toast for about 2 minutes. If you smell the chili powder starting to get a heavy, bitter aroma, take the pan off the heat immediately. Slowly stir about a cup of water into the pot until you have a semi-thick sauce. Add the remaining ingredients, bring to a simmer, and simmer for about 5 minutes. Puree the soup using an immersion blender, adding extra water as needed to achieve a thick but not pasty texture.

Options: If you use the chipotles and/or oregano, add them when you add the beans.

Per serving (½ of recipe): 344 calories, 19 g protein, 64 g carbohydrate, 2 g sugar, 3 g total fat, 6% calories from fat, 22 g fiber, 226 mg sodium

—JW

Curried Apple Daal Stew
Serves 2

The mustard seeds bring this soup to life, giving it a spicy, aromatic quality that heightens the sweetness of the apples.

½ onion, diced
1 tablespoon grated fresh ginger
2 teaspoons brown mustard seeds
1 tablespoon yellow curry powder
2½ cups water
¾ cup red lentils
2 green apples, cored and diced
3 tablespoons chopped fresh cilantro
¼ teaspoon sea salt
Optional: 1 roasted red bell pepper, diced, for garnish

Heat a medium saucepan over medium heat. Add the onion and cook until it softens, about 3 minutes. Add the ginger and mustard seeds and cook for 2 minutes. Stir in the curry powder. Immediately add the water and bring the mixture to a boil. Add the lentils, stir, and bring the liquid back to a boil. Cover the pan, reduce the heat to low, and cook for about 20 minutes. Remove from the heat and immediately stir in the apples, cilantro, and salt. Serve, garnished with the roasted bell pepper, if desired.

Tip: To keep the apples from browning, dice them at the very last minute before they go into the soup. Or, if you cut them up in advance, place them in a bowl with lots of cold water and a touch of lemon juice.

Per serving (½ of recipe): 424 calories, 22 g protein, 82 g carbohydrate, 21 g sugar, 3 g total fat, 7% calories from fat, 31 g fiber, 327 mg sodium

—*JW*

Ginger Lime Broth with Carrots and Rice Noodles

Serves 3

This soup leaves you feeling full but not heavy. It's perfect as a light meal or to serve alongside another dish.

4 cups water

2 tablespoons reduced-sodium soy sauce

2 tablespoons grated fresh ginger

Juice of 2 to 3 limes

1 stalk lemongrass, cut into 1-inch pieces and pressed with the flat of a knife

2 carrots, sliced

1 small bunch green onions, sliced

3 ounces rice noodles

Optional: ¼ cup light coconut milk; 8 ounces cubed extra-firm tofu

Combine the water and soy sauce in a large saucepan over medium-high heat and bring to a simmer. Add the ginger, lime juice, and lemongrass and simmer for 10 minutes. Add the carrots and green onions and simmer for another 5 minutes. Add the rice noodles and simmer until they are soft, about 2 minutes.

Options: If using the coconut milk and tofu, add them along with the carrots and green onions.

Per serving (⅓ of recipe): 184 calories, 2 g protein, 43 g carbohydrate, 5 g sugar, 0.4 g total fat, 2% calories from fat, 5 g fiber, 454 mg sodium

—JW

Salads

Mixed Greens and Spicy Roasted Tempeh
Serves 2

The spicy roasted tempeh makes this salad hearty and filling, while the Maple-Sage Dijon Dressing brings all the flavors together and makes the salad pop!

8 ounces tempeh, cut into bite-size squares
Pinch of ground allspice
Pinch of cayenne pepper
Pinch of ground cumin
1 small head red leaf lettuce, chopped
1½ cups chopped kale leaves
1 cup baby arugula
2 tomatoes, sliced
4 green onions, sliced
¼ cup Maple-Sage Dijon Dressing (page 217)

Preheat the oven to 375°F.

Place the tempeh cubes in a baking dish and spritz them with water. Add the allspice, cayenne, and cumin, and toss to coat. Cover the baking dish, place in the oven, and roast for 7 to 10 minutes.

Combine the lettuce, kale, arugula, tomatoes, and green onions in a salad bowl and toss with the dressing. Add the tempeh and toss to coat.

Per serving (½ of recipe): 319 calories, 30 g protein, 51 g carbohydrate, 37 g sugar, 6 g total fat, 16% calories from fat, 18 g fiber, 63 mg sodium

—JW

Salade Latine
Serves 2 as a main dish or 4 as a side dish

Swiss chard's slight bitterness is beautifully balanced by the sweetness of the corn and grapes, resulting in a surprising depth of flavor.

½ small white onion
3 cloves garlic

Leaves from 1 bunch Swiss chard
4 Roma tomatoes, diced
1½ cups fresh corn kernels
¼ cup pecan halves
1 cup seedless black grapes
Pinch of sea salt
½ teaspoon freshly ground black pepper

Mince the onion and garlic, then smash them together a couple of times with the back of a knife or with a mortar and pestle.

Wash the Swiss chard thoroughly, as it tends to be gritty, then slice it into ribbons by tightly bunching the leaves together and slicing them with a sharp, heavy knife. Place the Swiss chard in a salad bowl, add the remaining ingredients, and toss.

Per serving (½ of recipe): 181 calories, 7 g protein, 41 g carbohydrate, 17 g sugar, 2 g total fat, 9% calories from fat, 7 g fiber, 189 mg sodium

—JW

Rainbow Salad

Serves 2 as a main dish or 4 as a side dish

This delightful salad starts with sweet flavors, is topped with a berry dressing, and rounded out with some crisp greens.

1 head red leaf lettuce, shredded
1 large orange, peeled, pitted, and diced
1 cup seedless grapes
1 cup fresh blueberries
2 stalks celery, diced
½ teaspoon freshly ground white or black pepper
1 cup Strawberry Dressing (page 217)

Combine all the ingredients in a large salad bowl and toss until everything is well coated with dressing.

Per serving (½ of recipe): 249 calories, 10g protein, 60 g carbohydrate, 39 g sugar, 3 g total fat, 10% calories from fat, 17g fiber, 29 mg sodium

—JW

Easy Quinoa Tabouli Salad

Serves 4

A food processor makes this recipe a breeze!

4 cups low-sodium vegetable broth
2 cups quinoa, rinsed
Leaves from 1 bunch fresh parsley
1 small cucumber, seeded and cut into 1 x 2-inch pieces
½ cup sun-dried tomatoes (not packed in oil), soaked in water
   for 1 hour and drained
½ cup fresh lemon juice
Sea salt and freshly ground black pepper

Place the vegetable broth in a medium saucepan and bring to a boil over medium-high heat. Add the quinoa, cover, reduce the heat to low, and simmer for 20 minutes, or until the quinoa is fluffy and soft.

Meanwhile, combine the parsley, cucumber, and sun-dried tomatoes in a food processor and pulse until everything is chopped.

Transfer cooked quinoa to a large serving bowl, cool slightly, then add the chopped parsley mixture. Add the lemon juice and season with salt and pepper. Serve immediately, or refrigerate and serve chilled.

Per serving (¼ of recipe): 351 calories, 13 g protein, 64 g carbohydrate, 11 g sugar, 6 g total fat, 14% calories from fat, 8 g fiber, 378 mg sodium

—CW

Easy Colorful Pasta Salad

Serves 6

This quick lunch of yellow corn, green peas, orange carrots, and red kidney beans is almost too pretty to eat!

Salad:

4 cups cooked whole-grain spiral pasta
½ cup cooked corn kernels
½ cup cooked green peas

½ cup diced cooked carrots

1 cup cooked or canned low-sodium kidney beans, drained and rinsed

Dressing:

¼ cup maple syrup

¼ cup Dijon-style prepared mustard

1 tablespoon apple cider vinegar or vinegar of your choice

1½ tablespoons reduced-sodium soy sauce

1 tablespoon fresh orange juice

½ teaspoon garlic powder

1 teaspoon dried Italian seasoning

In a large bowl, combine all the salad ingredients.

To make the dressing, in a small bowl, combine all the ingredients and whisk together until well blended. Pour the dressing over the salad and stir gently. Adjust seasonings to taste, cover, and refrigerate for 1 hour before serving.

Tip: As a time-saver, use 1½ cups cooked mixed frozen vegetables in place of the fresh vegetables.

Per serving (⅙ of recipe): 230 calories, 9 g protein, 48 g carbohydrate, 11 g sugar, 1 g total fat, 5% calories from fat, 6 g fiber, 495 mg sodium

—CW

Black Bean Fiesta Salad

Serves 2

You can make this flavorful salad ahead of time, as it keeps for up to five days in the refrigerator.

2 cups cooked or canned low-sodium black beans, drained and rinsed

2 cups cooked corn kernels

¼ cup minced red onion

½ cup diced red bell pepper

3 green onions, thinly sliced

½ cup loosely packed fresh cilantro leaves, minced

¼ cup fresh lime juice
Sea salt and pepper to taste
Optional: Dash of cayenne pepper, or to taste

To make the salad, place all the ingredients in a large bowl and stir gently to combine. Cover and refrigerate for several hours before serving.

Per serving (½ of recipe): 394 calories, 21 g protein, 80 g carbohydrate, 13 g sugar, 2 g total fat, 5% calories from fat, 21 g fiber, 158 mg sodium

—CW

Brown Rice Salad

Serves 4 to 6

This whole-grain salad, with its variety of flavors and textures and antioxidant-rich colorful vegetables, is sure to satisfy.

1 cup quick-cooking brown rice
½ cup cooked or canned low-sodium garbanzo beans, drained and rinsed
½ cup shredded carrot
½ cup finely shredded red cabbage
¼ cup diced red bell pepper
¼ cup thinly sliced celery
¼ cup cooked green peas
¼ cup minced fresh parsley
1 tablespoon reduced-sodium soy sauce
3 tablespoons orange juice
1 teaspoon minced peeled fresh ginger

Cook the rice according to package directions.

In a large bowl, combine the cooked rice with the remaining ingredients. Adjust the seasonings to taste.

Per serving (¼ of recipe): 235 calories, 7 g protein, 47 g carbohydrate, 4 g sugar, 2 g total fat, 7% calories from fat, 7 g fiber, 169 mg sodium

—CW

Summer Salad

Serves 2 as a main dish or 4 as a side dish

The colors and textures will seduce you even before you taste this salad's sweet, cooling flavors. Because the flavor gets even better with time, it's perfectly portable.

½ red onion, diced

1 Mexican gray squash or zucchini, diced

1 cucumber, peeled and diced

2 small tomatoes, diced (and seeded if you like)

¼ cup sliced red cabbage

2 stalks celery, sliced

Kernels from 2 ears corn (about 1½ cups)

Pinch of sea salt

Juice of 1 small lime (about 1 tablespoon)

Optional: 3 tomatillos, diced; 2 tablespoons chopped fresh cilantro; 1 cup rinsed cooked or canned red beans or 1 cup sautéed tempeh; 1 cup sliced Swiss chard leaves

Mix all ingredients together in a large bowl and allow the salad to marinate for at least 30 minutes but preferably 2 hours. You can forgo this step and eat the salad right away, though the flavors won't be melded quite as much.

Options: If you use the tomatillos, peel away the papery part and make sure to wash them before cutting; this removes their sticky outer film and makes them much easier to handle. You can also use frozen corn in this recipe, though it will lack the crispness and sweetness of fresh corn. Want to make this a meal in itself instead of an accompaniment? Add the beans or tempeh and you'll have a delicious dinner in minutes.

Per serving (½ of recipe): 159 calories, 4 g protein, 36 g carbohydrate, 12 g sugar, 2 g total fat, 32% calories from fat, 7 g fiber, 246 mg sodium

—JW

Maple-Sage Dijon Dressing

Makes enough for 2 large salads (about ⅔ cup)

No doubt about it, the mustard, sage, and vinegar make this a potent dressing; the maple syrup sweetly balances it out. A little goes a long way. Try it on Mixed Greens and Spicy Roasted Tempeh (page 211) or the salad of your choice.

6 to 8 sage leaves
2 tablespoons low-sodium Dijon mustard
2 tablespoons low-sodium stone-ground mustard
1 tablespoon diced red onion
2 tablespoons red wine vinegar
3 tablespoons maple syrup

Crisp the sage leaves in a dry pan over medium-high heat for about 1 minute. Place all the ingredients in a blender and blend until smooth.

Per serving (½ of recipe): 187 calories, 1 g protein, 45 g carbohydrate, 16 g sugar, 1 g total fat, 5% calories from fat, 10 g fiber, 366 mg sodium

—JW

Strawberry Dressing

Makes enough for 1 large salad (about ⅔ cup)

Ginger gives this dressing a little bite, and the apple cider vinegar complements the flavor of the strawberries. Try it on the Rainbow Salad (page 212) or salad of your choice.

1 teaspoon grated fresh ginger
1 cup fresh or frozen and thawed strawberries
1 tablespoon apple cider vinegar

Place all the ingredients in a blender and blend until smooth.

Per serving: 49 calories, 1 g protein, 12 g carbohydrate, 1 g sugar, 0.5 g total fat, 9% calories from fat, 3 g fiber, 2 mg sodium

—Recipe by Madelyn Pryor

Sandwiches, Wraps, and Burgers

Garbanzo Bean Sandwiches

Makes 2 sandwiches

Here's a tasty and nutritious sandwich that's also high in protein.

1 15-ounce can low-sodium garbanzo beans, drained
2 tablespoons minced onion
1 small stalk celery, minced (about ¼ cup)
Freshly ground black pepper

Tofu mayo:

10 ounces low-fat silken tofu
½ teaspoon dry mustard
1 clove garlic, minced
¼ teaspoon sea salt, or to taste
1½ teaspoons apple cider vinegar
4 slices whole-grain bread, or 2 whole-grain pita pockets,
    cut in half
2 lettuce leaves or ½ cup alfalfa sprouts

Place the garbanzo beans in a large bowl and coarsely mash them
with a potato masher or fork. Add the onion and celery and set aside.

To make the tofu mayo, place the tofu, dry mustard, garlic, salt,
and vinegar in a food processor or blender and process until smooth.
Add the tofu mayo to the bean mixture and season with pepper to
taste. Mix well and serve on toasted whole-grain bread or tucked into
a pita pocket, with lettuce or sprouts.

Per serving (1 sandwich): 442 calories, 30 g protein, 67 g
carbohydrate, 8 g sugar, 7 g total fat, 14% calories from fat, 13 g
fiber, 699 mg sodium

—CW

Baked Veggie Falafel

Serves 4

Falafel is a popular Middle Eastern food made from garbanzo beans. This easy, fat-free version is baked instead of fried!

  1 15-ounce can low-sodium garbanzo beans, drained and rinsed
  2 tablespoons minced onion
  1 clove garlic, minced
  1 tablespoon minced fresh parsley
  ¼ cup shredded carrot
  1 tablespoon fresh lemon juice
  2 tablespoons whole-wheat pastry flour
  1 teaspoon ground coriander seeds
  1 teaspoon ground cumin
  ¼ cup cooked green peas
  Sea salt and freshly ground black pepper

Preheat the oven to 350°F and lightly oil a baking sheet.

Place the garbanzo beans, onion, garlic, parsley, carrot, lemon juice, flour, coriander, and cumin in a food processor and process until fairly smooth. Transfer the mixture to a medium bowl and stir in the peas. Season with salt and pepper to taste.

Form the mixture into 8 patties and place them on the prepared baking sheet. Bake for 15 minutes, then carefully turn the patties over and bake for 15 more minutes. Serve 2 patties stuffed inside a whole-wheat pita pocket. Top with a little hummus, shredded lettuce, and diced onion and tomato. The patties also are great served with couscous and a salad.

Per serving (¼ of recipe): 149 calories, 8 g protein, 26 g carbohydrate, 1 g sugar, 2 g total fat, 12% calories from fat, 6 g fiber, 214 mg sodium

—CW

Portobello Burgers

Serves 4

These burgers are fast and easy to make. Enjoy them on whole-grain buns with your favorite toppings.

   4 portobello mushroom caps
   1 tablespoon reduced-sodium soy sauce
   Freshly ground black pepper
   4 whole-grain burger buns
   Optional toppings: ketchup, mustard, sliced red onion, and lettuce
      or sprouts

Preheat the oven to 400°F.

Use a spoon to scrape the gills off the mushrooms and discard the gills. Place the mushrooms stem side down on a baking sheet and lightly brush each with some of the soy sauce. Sprinkle with a little black pepper.

Place in the oven and bake for 10 to 15 minutes, until tender. Serve on the buns, topped with any or all of the toppings.

   Per serving (1 burger): 125 calories, 8 g protein, 21 g carbohydrate, 6 g sugar, 2 g total fat, 13% calories from fat, 4 g fiber, 434 mg sodium

—CW

Tuscan Wrap

Serves 2

This simple white bean and sun-dried tomato spread makes an excellent cheese alternative and can be eaten as a dip in its own right. But why not add some shredded veggies and wrap it up for a lovely lunch, like we've done here?

   2 cups cooked or canned low-sodium white kidney (cannellini)
      beans, drained and rinsed
   1 clove garlic
   1 teaspoon minced fresh rosemary
   ½ teaspoon freshly ground pepper
   8 to 10 sun-dried tomatoes (not packed in oil), soaked in water
      and drained

1 zucchini, shredded
1 carrot, shredded
1 cup sprouts
2 whole-wheat tortillas

Combine the beans, garlic, rosemary, pepper, and sun-dried tomatoes in a blender and blend into a thick paste.

Spread the bean dip on the tortillas, top with the zucchini, carrot, and sprouts, and roll them up to make wraps.

Per serving (1 wrap): 373 calories, 24 g protein, 78 g carbohydrate, 13 g sugar, 2 g total fat, 4% calories from fat, 17 g fiber, 497 mg sodium

—JW

Garden Pita Wrap

Serves 1

This makes a huge wrap! The best way to have this is wrapped or folded in a large pita, but a tortilla will do in a pinch.

3 or 4 cauliflower florets
1 carrot, sliced
3 or 4 broccoli florets
¼ onion, sliced
1 tomato, chopped
2 cloves garlic, minced
2 teaspoons reduced-sodium tamari
½ cup cooked brown rice
¼ cup cooked or canned low-sodium red beans, drained and rinsed
1 whole-wheat pita or tortilla
Hot sauce (such as Sriracha or habanero)

Heat a medium skillet over high heat. Add the cauliflower, carrot, broccoli, and onion and cook for about 5 to 7 minutes, until they just start to brown. Reduce the heat to medium, add the tomato, garlic, and tamari, and cook for 1 more minute. Place the rice and beans on the pita and add the vegetable mixture.

Tip: This wrap is great with raw veggies, too. Sprinkle the tamari into the rice, as you won't be cooking it with the veggies.

Per serving: 487 calories, 22 g protein, 103 g carbohydrate, 11 g sugar, 2 g total fat, 4% calories from fat, 15 g fiber, 687 mg sodium

—JW

Wild Mushroom Lettuce Wraps
Serves 2

This is a delicious wrap, and it is also a great example of how you can mix and match ingredients. If you don't have bok choy, you can use cabbage. If you don't have water chestnuts, you can use sliced carrots for crunch. If you don't have bean sprouts, you can instead add noodles to the stir-fry portion of the recipe. The key ingredients are the mushrooms, green onions, and tamari. Everything else is negotiable.

2 heads baby bok choy, thinly sliced

8 to 10 fresh shiitake mushrooms, thickly sliced

½ cup roughly chopped oyster mushrooms

6 to 8 green onions, sliced

2 cloves garlic, minced

3 tablespoons diced water chestnuts

¼ teaspoon Chinese five-spice powder or ¼ teaspoon freshly ground black pepper and a pinch of cloves

2 teaspoons reduced-sodium tamari or soy sauce

½ teaspoon chili paste

½ cup bean sprouts

¼ cup chopped enoki mushrooms

4 lettuce leaves (preferably butterleaf lettuce)

Optional: 1 teaspoon grated fresh ginger

Optional sauce: 3 tablespoons hoisin sauce mixed with 2 tablespoons water

Heat a wok or a wide, shallow sauté pan over high heat. Add the bok choy and cook for 30 seconds. Add the shiitake mushrooms and cook for another 30 seconds. Add the oyster mushrooms, green onions, garlic, and water chestnuts and cook for another minute. Add the Chinese five-spice and stir. Immediately stir in the tamari or soy sauce. Stir in the chili paste and cook for another 15 seconds. Remove from the heat and immediately add the bean sprouts and enoki mushrooms. Serve in the lettuce leaves.

Options: Add the ginger when you add the garlic and serve the wraps with the hoisin dipping sauce.

Per serving (1 wrap): 90 calories, 6 g protein, 14 g carbohydrate, 4 g sugar, 1 g total fat, 29% calories from fat, 6 g fiber, 192 mg sodium

—JW

Tacos with Potatoes, Swiss Chard, and Pinto Beans
Serves 2

South of the border, tacos have a surprising diversity that encompasses greens, beans, potatoes, a plethora of peppers, grilled veggies, and succulent sauces.

½ yellow onion, sliced

2 cloves garlic, minced

1 red potato, chopped

1 cup sliced Swiss chard leaves

1 chipotle chile in adobo, minced (substitute ¼ green bell pepper if you can't handle the heat)

¼ teaspoon sea salt

Almond milk or water

1 cup cooked or canned low-sodium pinto beans, drained and rinsed

4 corn tortillas, warmed

Chimichurri Sauce (page 244), for topping

Heat a medium skillet over medium-high heat. Add the onion and cook for about 5 to 6 minutes, until it starts to brown. Add the garlic, potato, Swiss chard, chipotle, and salt. Add a thin layer (about ¼ inch) of almond milk, bring to a simmer, and simmer, keeping that ¼ inch of liquid in the pan, until the potatoes are just starting to soften. Now cook out as much of the liquid as possible without turning the potatoes mushy (better to leave a bit of liquid than have mushy potatoes!). Remove the pan from the heat and immediately stir in the beans. Divide the filling among the tortillas and top with Chimichurri Sauce. If you'd like to make tostadas, use flat tortillas.

Tip: Corn tortillas should be warmed before serving so that they're pliable. You can steam the tortillas for 2 to 3 minutes or spritz them with water and warm them in a dry pan over medium heat for about 1 minute per side. This keeps the tortillas from falling apart when you fold them.

Per serving (½ of recipe): 300 calories, 13 g protein, 60 g carbohydrate, 4 g sugar, 2 g total fat, 6% calories from fat, 13 g fiber, 353 mg sodium

—*JW*

Tortas Frijoles

Serves 2

The torta is a quintessential Mexican sandwich. This particular torta is done in the style of Jalisco, featuring a bun filled with beans and onions and drowned in a spicy tomato pepper sauce. For a milder flavor, omit the chili powder.

½ yellow onion, thinly sliced; or ¼ cup pickled onion slices

2 tablespoons chili powder

2 cups canned crushed fire-roasted tomatoes

1 tablespoon white wine vinegar

¼ teaspoon salt

1½ cups vegetarian refried beans, warmed

2 bolillo rolls or hoagie rolls, cut in half and toasted

Heat a small skillet over medium-high heat. Add the onion and cook for about 8 to 10 minutes, until it is heavily browned. Give the pan a splash of water and stir quickly. Once the water evaporates, in about 15 seconds, remove the pan from the heat.

In a small saucepan, toast the chili powder for about 1 minute, then add the fire-roasted tomatoes, vinegar, and salt and heat until the tomatoes are warmed through. Remove from the heat, spread the beans over the bottom half of each sandwich roll, and top with the onions. Pour the sauce over the top (or serve it on the side as a dipping sauce) and top with the bottom half of the rolls.

Per serving (1 torta): 532 calories, 26 g protein, 104 g carbohydrate, 13 g sugar, 4 g total fat, 6% calories from fat, 22 g fiber, 816 mg sodium

—*JW*

Grilled Eggplant Niçoise
Serves 4

This simple Mediterranean sandwich makes an elegant lunch or a late-afternoon dinner.

    4 cloves garlic
    1 large eggplant, sliced into thick slabs
    Juice of 4 lemons (about ½ cup)
    ¼ teaspoon cracked black pepper
    1 tablespoon dried lavender
    ½ teaspoon saffron
    4 large slices French bread or sourdough bread, toasted
    1 small fennel bulb, sliced
    2 tomatoes, sliced
    ¼ cup sliced pitted Niçoise olives or green olives

Smash the garlic and rub each slab of eggplant with the garlic. Place the eggplant in a shallow bowl and pour the lemon juice over it. Add enough water to submerge the eggplant. Allow the eggplant to marinate for at least 1 hour, then drain and place it in a shallow dish. Add the garlic, pepper, lavender, and saffron and let it sit for about 1 hour.

Place the eggplant directly on a grill over medium heat and cook until it is soft on both sides but not charred. Place a grilled slab of eggplant on a slice of bread and top with a couple of slices of fennel and tomatoes and about 1 tablespoon sliced olives. This sandwich is served open-faced.

Per serving (1 sandwich): 154 calories, 7 g protein, 35 g carbohydrate, 9 g sugar, 2 g total fat, 9% calories from fat, 10 g fiber, 478 mg sodium

—JW

Main Dishes

English Muffin Pizzas

Serves 2 to 4

These fun little pizzas using healthful ingredients make a fast meal.

4 whole-wheat English muffins, split
½ cup canned low-sodium pizza sauce
¼ cup cooked broccoli florets
¼ cup thinly sliced mushrooms
¼ cup drained, rinsed, and chopped roasted red bell pepper

Preheat the oven to 375°F.

Place the English muffins on a baking sheet. Spoon some of the pizza sauce onto each muffin. Top with a little broccoli, mushrooms, and roasted red pepper, evenly dividing the toppings among the English muffins. Bake for 10 minutes and serve hot.

Per serving (¼ of recipe): 158 calories, 7 g protein, 31 g carbohydrate, 6 g sugar, 2 g total fat, 10% calories from fat, 6 g fiber, 371 mg sodium

—*CW*

Easy Black Bean Skillet

Serves 4

This superfast recipe uses canned beans and minute brown rice as a time-saver.

1 cup diced onion
½ cup diced green bell pepper
2 cloves garlic, minced
1 teaspoon dried oregano
1 15-ounce can low-sodium black beans, drained and rinsed
1 cup diced fresh or canned tomatoes
1 cup low-sodium vegetable broth
1½ cups uncooked minute brown rice
Sea salt and freshly ground black pepper

Menus and Recipes 227

1 tablespoon minced fresh cilantro
Optional: hot sauce

Heat 2 tablespoons water in a large skillet over medium heat. Add
the onion, bell pepper, garlic, and oregano. Cook, stirring, for
5 minutes, or until the onion is translucent. Add the beans, tomatoes,
and vegetable broth and bring to a boil. Add the rice and stir well.
Cover, reduce the heat to low, and simmer for 5 minutes. Season with
salt and pepper to taste and simmer for 3 more minutes.

Remove from the heat and let sit for 5 minutes, then sprinkle with
the cilantro and serve, with hot sauce, if desired.

Per serving (¼ of recipe): 391 calories, 13 g protein, 80 g carbohydrate,
5 g sugar, 3 g total fat, 6% calories from fat, 15 g fiber, 538 mg sodium

—CW

Mexican Polenta Casserole

Serves 4

This hearty casserole is a real crowd-pleaser.

- 1 16-ounce package precooked polenta (plain, mushroom and onion, or other flavor)
- 1 cup diced onion
- ½ cup chopped green bell pepper
- 1 cup thinly sliced carrots
- 1 teaspoon ground cumin
- 1½ teaspoons dried cilantro
- 2 tablespoons whole-wheat pastry flour
- ¾ cup low-sodium vegetable broth
- 1 cup frozen corn kernels
- 2 cups cooked or canned low-sodium pinto beans, drained and rinsed

Preheat the oven to 375°F and lightly oil an 8 x 11-inch Pyrex baking
dish.

Mash the polenta and spread it over the prepared baking dish,
pressing down gently and evenly.

Heat 2 tablespoons water in a medium skillet over medium
heat and add the onion, bell pepper, carrots, cumin, and cilantro.

Cook, stirring, for about 5 minutes. Add the flour and stir until the vegetables are well coated. Cook for 1 to 2 minutes, stirring constantly. Slowly add the vegetable broth and cook for 5 minutes, or until the mixture is thick and bubbly. Stir in the corn kernels and beans and heat them through.

Pour the vegetable-bean mixture evenly over the polenta. Cover, place in the oven, and bake for 30 minutes, or until bubbly. Remove from the oven, uncover, and let sit for 10 to 15 minutes before slicing and serving. Serve with a fresh garden salad.

Per serving (¼ of recipe): 271 calories, 12 g protein, 56 g carbohydrate, 5 g sugar, 2 g total fat, 5% calories from fat, 11 g fiber, 346 mg sodium

—CW

Sweet Potato Burritos

Serves 4

Sweet meets spicy in these nutritious and tasty burritos.

2 cups peeled and diced sweet potatoes
1 cup frozen corn kernels
1 15-ounce can low-sodium black beans, drained and rinsed
1 teaspoon very thinly sliced green onion
1 tablespoon fresh lime juice
1 teaspoon chili powder
Sea salt and freshly ground black pepper
4 8-inch whole-wheat tortillas, warmed
1 cup prepared salsa
2 cups shredded lettuce

Place the sweet potatoes in a medium saucepan and add water to come an inch up the sides. Place over medium-high heat and bring to a boil; cook for 5 minutes, or until the sweet potatoes are tender. Add the corn and cook 1 more minute.

Drain and transfer to a large bowl. Add the black beans, green onion, lime juice, and chili powder; season with salt and pepper to taste. Divide the filling among the tortillas, top with the salsa and lettuce, roll them up, and serve.

Per serving (1 burrito): 298 calories, 13 g protein, 62 g carbohydrate, 8 g sugar, 2 g total fat, 7% calories from fat, 15 g fiber, 891 mg sodium

—*CW*

Baked Ziti

Serves 4

The ultimate classic casserole goes low fat! This dish is delicious and light.

½ teaspoon olive oil

8 ounces uncooked whole-grain ziti or penne pasta

10.5 ounces firm low-fat tofu, drained

2 tablespoons whole-wheat pastry flour

1 teaspoon garlic powder

1 teaspoon onion powder

1 teaspoon dried basil

½ teaspoon dried oregano

½ teaspoon sea salt, or to taste

1 24-ounce jar fat-free spaghetti sauce

Optional: ½ cup cooked chopped Swiss chard, mushrooms, or zucchini

Preheat the oven to 375°F and grease a 2½-quart casserole dish with the oil.

Cook the pasta according to the package directions to al dente.

Crumble the drained tofu into a bowl and add the flour, garlic powder, onion powder, basil, oregano, and salt. Mix well. Gently fold in the cooked pasta, spaghetti sauce, and any optional ingredients.

Spoon the pasta-tofu mixture into the prepared casserole dish and bake for 25 minutes or until firm and lightly golden on top. Serve hot with a fresh garden salad.

Per serving (¼ of recipe): 237 calories, 12 g protein, 42 g carbohydrate, 9 g sugar, 4 g total fat, 14% calories from fat, 6 g fiber, 556 mg sodium

—*CW*

Spaghetti with White Bean Marinara Sauce
Serves 4

Adding beans to your spaghetti sauce makes it hearty and satisfying, not to mention higher in protein and fiber, making this a winning recipe for both taste and nutrition! A side of steamed kale or broccoli completes the meal.

10 ounces uncooked whole-grain spaghetti
1 24-ounce jar fat-free spaghetti sauce
1 15-ounce can low-sodium cannellini beans, drained and rinsed

Cook the spaghetti according to the package directions; drain.

Meanwhile, in a medium saucepan, combine the spaghetti sauce and beans, cover, and warm over low heat. Serve the spaghetti topped with the marinara-bean mixture.

Per serving (¼ of recipe): 403 calories, 18 g protein, 85 g carbohydrate, 14 g sugar, 1 g total fat, 3% calories from fat, 11 g fiber, 655 mg sodium

—CW

Veggie Kebabs
Serves 4

Serve these savory kebabs over a brown rice pilaf for a satisfying and easy meal.

16 cherry tomatoes
2 red onions, each cut into 8 bite-size chunks
2 green or red bell peppers, cored, seeded, and cut into 8 pieces each
16 button mushrooms
1 small yellow summer squash, cut into 8 pieces
1 small zucchini, cut into 8 pieces

Marinade:

½ cup balsamic vinegar
½ cup orange juice
2 tablespoons maple syrup
2 tablespoons prepared mustard

1 teaspoon dried Italian seasoning

½ teaspoon sea salt

¼ teaspoon ground black pepper

8 metal skewers, or bamboo skewers soaked in water for
   30 minutes

Place the cherry tomatoes, red onions, bell peppers, mushrooms, squash, and zucchini in a large bowl.

In a small bowl, combine the marinade ingredients and whisk well. Pour the marinade over the vegetables and stir to coat. Marinate for 15 minutes.

Heat a charcoal or gas grill or your oven's broiler. Onto one skewer, thread the ingredients in the following manner: 1 tomato, 1 red onion chunk, 1 pepper piece, 1 mushroom, 1 yellow summer squash slice, 1 tomato, 1 zucchini slice, 1 red onion chunk, 1 pepper, and 1 mushroom. Repeat with remaining ingredients and skewers. Place the kebabs on the hot grill or a broiler pan and brush with the marinade. Grill for 7 minutes, or until desired tenderness, turning the kebabs a few times. Serve immediately.

Per serving (2 kebabs): 110 calories, 4 g protein, 24 g carbohydrate, 14 g sugar, 0.9 g total fat, 7% calories from fat, 4 g fiber, 206 mg sodium

—CW

Risotto Primavera
Serves 4

This version of primavera uses nutritious brown rice to make a creamy easy-to-prepare dish.

1 cup diced onion

2 cloves garlic, minced

1 cup sliced mushrooms

½ cup diced red bell pepper

½ cup diced carrot

1 cup uncooked short-grain brown rice, rinsed

4 cups low-sodium vegetable broth

½ cup green peas

½ cup asparagus, ends trimmed and cut into ½-inch pieces
½ cup diced yellow summer squash
¼ cup minced fresh parsley

Preheat oven to 350°F.

Heat 2 tablespoons water in a Dutch oven or large, deep skillet over medium heat. Add the onion and garlic and cook, stirring, for 5 minutes. Add the mushrooms, bell pepper, and carrot and cook, stirring, for another 5 minutes. Stir in the rice and cook for 2 more minutes. Add the broth, increase the heat to medium-high, and bring to a boil. If using an ovenproof pan, cover the pan and transfer to the oven. If using a skillet that is not ovenproof, pour the rice mixture into a very lightly oiled 2-quart casserole and transfer to the oven. Bake, covered, for 1 hour.

Meanwhile, steam the green peas, asparagus, and squash together until crisp-tender, about 3 to 5 minutes. Remove the risotto from the oven and fold in the steamed vegetables. Serve hot, garnished with the parsley.

Time-saving tip: Use frozen diced vegetables in place of fresh if you are short on time.

Per serving (¼ of recipe): 233 calories, 7 g protein, 49 g carbohydrate, 8 g sugar, 2 g total fat, 6% calories from fat, 7 g fiber, 973 mg sodium

—CW

Gnocchi with Basil and Sun-dried Tomatoes
Serves 2

Gnocchi is simple and elegant and needs few other ingredients to make it shine.

4 to 6 basil leaves, sliced into ribbons
1½ cups dairy-free whole-wheat gnocchi
10 to 12 sun-dried tomatoes
1 teaspoon cracked black pepper

Lay the basil leaves on top of one another, roll them up, and slice them into ribbons.

Bring a medium saucepan of water to a boil. Add the gnocchi and stir; cook until the gnocchi float. Remove them as they come to the top of the water and drain. Transfer to a serving bowl and toss the gnocchi with the basil ribbons, sun-dried tomatoes, and pepper and serve.

Make your own gnocchi! Boil 2 pounds of Yukon gold potatoes or sweet potatoes until they are soft, about 45 minutes. Once the potatoes come out of the water, peel them as best you can, but be careful because they'll be quite hot (peeling just after cooking prevents the water absorption that occurs when peeled potatoes are boiled). Mash the potatoes, add ¾ cup whole-wheat pastry flour and ¼ teaspoon salt to the potatoes, and gently mix until the ingredients are thoroughly incorporated. Gently knead the dough until it doesn't stick to your fingers but is still soft. If it is too moist, you may need to incorporate up to ¼ cup more flour. Roll the dough into cigar shapes and slice the rolls into 1-inch pieces. Boil the gnocchi until they float, which will take only about 1 minute. Making gnocchi takes a little practice, but it's worth it.

Per serving (½ of recipe): 211 calories, 5 g protein, 48 g carbohydrate, 6 g sugar, 0.4 g total fat, 2% calories from fat, 3 g fiber, 714 mg sodium

—JW

Asian Stir-Fry with Apricot Teriyaki Sauce

Serves 4

Serve this sweet and savory stir-fry over a bed of brown rice or quinoa for a winning dinner!

¼ cup low-sodium vegetable broth

½ cup all-fruit apricot preserves

1 tablespoon reduced-sodium soy sauce

1 teaspoon rice vinegar

1 teaspoon cornstarch

1 cup onion sliced into half-moons

2 cloves garlic, minced

4 cups halved button mushrooms

1 cup carrots cut into matchsticks

1 cup shredded green cabbage

2 cups broccoli spears

1 cup yellow summer squash sliced into half-moons

In a small bowl, whisk together the vegetable broth, preserves, soy sauce, vinegar, and cornstarch. Set aside.

In a wok or large skillet, heat 2 tablespoons water over medium-high heat. Add the onion and garlic and cook, stirring, for 5 minutes. Add the mushrooms and cook for 2 more minutes. Add the carrots and cabbage and cook for another 2 minutes. Add the broccoli and squash and cook just until they are crisp-tender, about 2 minutes. Pour the sauce over the vegetables and gently stir; cook until the sauce thickens slightly. Serve immediately.

Time-saving tip: Use 1 16-ounce package frozen stir-fry vegetable blend in place of fresh vegetables.

Per serving (¼ of recipe): 162 calories, 5 g protein, 38 g carbohydrate, 23 g sugar, 0.7 g total fat, 4% calories from fat, 7 g fiber, 315 mg sodium

—CW

Stuffed Peppers with Squash, Black Beans, and Rice
Serves 2 as a main dish or 4 as a side dish

If you have leftover rice and cooked black beans on hand, this recipe can be made in just a few minutes. Or you can slice up the red peppers, add some shredded lettuce, and make a salad out of it!

½ cup cooked brown rice

1 cup cooked black beans

2 Mexican gray squash or zucchini, diced

6 green onions, sliced

2 teaspoons pepitas (green pumpkin seeds)

2 cloves garlic, minced

1 tablespoon chopped fresh oregano

2 tablespoons apple cider vinegar

Juice of 1 lime

¼ teaspoon sea salt

½ teaspoon freshly ground black pepper

2 red bell peppers, cut in half, cored, and seeded

Optional: salsa

Combine the rice, beans, squash, green onions, pepitas, garlic, oregano, vinegar, lime, salt, and pepper in a large bowl. Fill the pepper halves with the squash, rice, and bean mixture. Top with salsa, if desired, and serve.

Per serving (½ of stuffed pepper): 187 calories, 16 g protein, 54 g carbohydrate, 13 g sugar, 3 g total fat, 14% calories from fat, 16 g fiber, 317 mg sodium

—*JW*

Sides

Toasted Brown Rice

Makes 3 cups

Brown rice is delicious when you learn the cooking secrets in this simple recipe. By toasting it first, then cooking it like pasta, it comes out absolutely perfect.

1 cup short-grain brown rice

3 cups water

In a saucepan, rinse the rice briefly with water, then pour off as much of the water as you can. You are now left with damp rice.

Place the pan over high heat and stir the rice until dry, 1 to 2 minutes. Add the water, bring to a boil, then reduce the heat and simmer for about 40 minutes, until the rice is thoroughly cooked but still has a touch of crunchiness. Drain off any remaining water (do not cook it until all the water is absorbed).

To serve, top with sunflower or sesame seeds, soy sauce, or whatever you like.

Per ½-cup serving: 115 calories, 3 g protein, 24 g carbohydrate, 0.4 g sugar, 0.9 g fat, 7% calories from fat, 3 g fiber, 5 mg sodium

Red Rice

Serves 4

This is the Mexican version of Spanish rice and really deserves the roasted peppers in the option section! With a cup of beans, you can make this into a meal.

½ yellow onion, chopped

4 Roma tomatoes (or 8 tomatillos), chopped

1¼ cups water

1 teaspoon white vinegar

½ teaspoon sea salt

1 cup brown rice

Optional: 1 diced roasted Hatch or poblano chile; or
    2 to 3 tablespoons diced roasted green chiles

Heat a medium saucepan over medium heat; add the onion and cook until it is translucent, about 3 to 4 minutes, stirring every 30 seconds or so. Add the tomatoes, water, vinegar, and salt and bring to a simmer. Add the rice and return to a simmer. Cover, reduce the heat to low, and cook for about 25 minutes.

Options: Add the roasted pepper along with the tomatoes. If you prefer to roast your own chiles instead of using the canned version, place the chiles in a dry skillet over medium-high heat and toast until the side touching the pan is almost completely blistered. Flip the peppers and toast on the other side. Cool enough to handle, then peel as much of the blistered part of the skin away from the peppers as possible. The flatter your peppers, the more success you will have with this method.

Per serving (¼ of recipe): 182 calories, 4 g protein, 38 g carbohydrate, 2 g sugar, 1 g total fat, 7% calories from fat, 2 g fiber, 146 mg sodium

—JW

Six Ways to Cook Sweet Potatoes

Sweet potatoes are one of the most healthful foods ever to pop out of the ground. Loaded with beta-carotene and naturally sweet, they are practically a meal all by themselves. There are countless ways to cook them; here are six very easy ones:

Boiled. Peel the sweet potatoes, cut into chunks, toss into boiling water, and cook until soft, about 20 minutes. Drain and mash with a fork or immersion blender. If you like, stir in some orange juice or brown sugar, or top with cinnamon.

Steamed. Cut the sweet potatoes into 2-inch chunks and steam for about 5 minutes in a steamer basket. Season with cumin, chili powder, and fresh cilantro. Mash and serve over rice.

Another way to season them is to whisk together 2 tablespoons vegan mayonnaise, the juice of 1 lime, and 1½ teaspoons curry powder; stir into the sweet potatoes and top with chopped fresh cilantro.

Baked. Wet and pierce the skin with a fork, then place on a baking sheet or in an ovenproof pan and bake at 350°F for about 40 minutes. Season with a little salt and pepper.

As an extra-moist and delicious alternative, preheat the oven to 450°F. Place the sweet potatoes directly on an oven rack, with foil or a baking sheet below to catch drips. Do not poke holes into the sweet potatoes. Bake for 20 minutes, then reduce the temperature to 350°F and bake for an additional 60 minutes.

And here's a way to get really fancy: Peel and slice 1 or 2 sweet potatoes into ½-inch rounds and place in a baking dish. Whisk together ¼ cup seasoned rice vinegar, 2 tablespoons low-sodium soy sauce, and 1 teaspoon dried oregano or rosemary and pour over the top. Cover with foil and bake for 20 minutes at 400°F. Remove the foil and bake for another 10 minutes.

Roasted. Cut into 2-inch cubes. Roast at 450°F alone or with onions, Brussels sprouts, or other root vegetables.

Microwaved. Pierce sweet potatoes all over with a fork, then place in the microwave, jackets and all. Cover with a paper towel and microwave on high for 3 to 4 minutes. Turn them over and microwave for an additional 3 to 4 minutes. Top with a little salt and pepper, or perhaps chopped walnuts or dates, raisins, or cinnamon. They also go well with salsa or hummus.

Slow-cooked. Wash the sweet potatoes, but do not dry them, and fill a slow cooker with as many as it can hold. There is no need to poke holes in them or add any cooking liquid. Just cook on low for about 7 hours, until tender. Cut open and enjoy them plain, or remove the skins and mash them.

And did you know that you can use sweet potatoes as a thickener when making soup? They go especially well in broccoli soup and chili.

Per medium sweet potato: 103 calories, 2 g protein, 24 g carbohydrate, 7 g sugar, 0.2 g total fat, 1% of calories from fat, 4 g fiber, 41 mg sodium

Moroccan Mint Couscous

Serves 3

Moroccan mint tea, a gunpowder tea (meaning the leaves have been rolled into pellets) flavored with lots of mint, suffuses the couscous, giving it a full-bodied taste, which is balanced by sweet apricots, spicy chile paste, and salty olives.

¾ cup hot mint tea

¾ cup uncooked couscous

4 to 5 dried apricots, chopped

8 to 10 pitted dried black olives or pitted whole kalamata olives

1 tablespoon chile paste, preferably harissa sauce

½ cup cooked chickpeas, drained and rinsed

Combine the hot tea and couscous in a medium bowl. As the couscous absorbs the liquid, slowly fluff it with a fork. Add the remaining ingredients, stir together, and serve.

Per serving (⅓ of recipe): 404 calories, 14 g protein, 19 g carbohydrate, 11 g sugar, 3 g total fat, 11% calories from fat, 9 g fiber, 258 mg sodium

—JW

That Delish Potato Dish

Serves 10 (makes 10 cups)

This dish really wows people and couldn't be simpler. It goes especially well with steamed broccoli and a salad.

3 carrots, peeled and sliced ½ inch thick

1 medium to large sweet potato, peeled and cut into 1-inch pieces

6 small red potatoes, cut into 1-inch pieces

1 medium red onion, quartered and sliced

1 medium yellow onion, quartered and sliced

3 tablespoons reduced-sodium soy sauce

3 tablespoons Bragg Liquid Aminos

¼ cup water

1 teaspoon garlic powder (no salt added)

½ teaspoon Italian seasoning (no salt added)

Preheat the oven to 350°F and lightly spray an 11 x 13-inch baking pan with cooking spray.

Place the vegetables in the prepared baking dish and toss to mix. Whisk together the soy sauce, liquid aminos, water, garlic powder, and Italian seasoning and pour over the vegetables. Cover tightly with foil and bake for 1½ hours. Stir the vegetables and serve.

Per 1-cup serving: 66 calories, 2 g protein, 15 g carbohydrate, 0.1 g total fat, 2% calories from fat, 2 g fiber, 327 mg sodium

—Recipe from Riva Gebel

Plantains in Cumin Tomato Sauce
Serves 2

East African cuisine has long been influenced by India, but it has a more rustic, hearty feel to it.

1½ teaspoons cumin seeds
1 tablespoon coriander seeds
½ onion, sliced
1 red bell pepper, cored, seeded, and diced
3 cloves garlic, minced
4 Roma tomatoes, chopped, or 12 ounces crushed tomatoes
¼ teaspoon sea salt
3 plantains, sliced in half lengthwise and cut into 3-inch strips
Optional: 1 diced jalapeño; ¼ teaspoon ground turmeric;
    1 cup chopped collard greens; 2 tablespoons chopped
    peanuts

Toast the cumin seeds and coriander seeds in a large dry sauté pan over medium heat until the coriander seeds start to pop, about 1½ minutes. Add the onion and bell pepper and cook for about 4 or 5 minutes, until the onion starts to brown. Add the garlic and cook for 1 more minute. Add the tomatoes and salt and continue cooking until the tomatoes reduce to a sauce. Add the plantains and simmer until they are cooked but not mushy, adding water to the pan every so often to make sure the sauce halfway covers the plantains.

Options: If you use the jalapeño, add it along with the tomatoes.
Same with the turmeric and collard greens. The turmeric will give this
dish a tangy curry flavor, and the collard greens will pair naturally
with the cumin tomato sauce. The peanuts are used as a garnish for
the finished dish.

Per serving (½ of recipe): 398 calories, 6 g protein, 101 g carbohydrate,
48 g sugar, 2 g total fat, 5% calories from fat, 12 g fiber, 301 mg sodium

—JW

East African Quinoa Pilaf
Serves 3

Pilaf, or pilau, is usually made with rice, but the nutty flavor of quinoa
is an excellent canvas for the colors of the East African spices.

- 1¼ cups quinoa
- 1 red onion, diced
- 1 carrot, diced
- 1 tablespoon coriander seeds
- 1 teaspoon cumin seeds
- 2 cloves garlic, minced
- 2 teaspoons minced ginger
- 1 serrano chile, minced (substitute ½ to 1 jalapeño for less heat)
- 3 Roma tomatoes, chopped
- 1 cup sliced collard greens (or kale or mustard greens), stripped
  from stems
- ½ teaspoon ground cardamom
- ½ teaspoon ground cinnamon
- ¼ teaspoon sea salt
- Optional: 2 tablespoons slivered almonds

Steam the quinoa for 20 minutes using a steamer with reasonably
small holes (don't worry if some quinoa falls through into the water).

Heat a medium sauté pan over medium heat. Add the onion and
carrot and cook until they are just soft, about 3 minutes. Add the
coriander and cumin seeds and cook for about 1 minute. Add the
garlic, ginger, and chile and cook for 1 minute. Add the tomatoes,
collard greens, cardamom, cinnamon, and salt and cook for about

5 minutes, until the collard greens are just tender. Stir in the steamed quinoa and slivered almonds, if desired.

Per serving: 324 calories, 15.6 g protein, 62 g carbohydrate, 4 g sugar, 5 g total fat, 14% calories from fat, 9 g fiber, 334 mg sodium

—JW

Sauces

Cream Gravy
Makes about 1 cup

This is a healthy version of the cream gravy often used in the South. The flavor comes not from milk and fat but from pepper and other spices.

- 3 tablespoons whole-wheat flour (preferably whole-wheat pastry flour)
- ⅛ teaspoon sea salt
- ½ to 1 teaspoon cracked black pepper
- 1 cup unsweetened soy milk or almond milk
- Optional: 1 teaspoon fresh chopped rosemary; 1 clove minced garlic; ¼ teaspoon crushed red pepper; 1 teaspoon grated nutmeg; or ½ minced onion

Heat a wide saucepan over medium heat. Add the flour, salt, and pepper and toast, stirring, for about 2 minutes, until the flour develops a nutty aroma. Slowly stir in the soy milk about ¼ cup at a time, thoroughly incorporating each addition of liquid before moving on to the next. Simmer the gravy for about 5 minutes. If it gets lumpy, put it in a blender and blend for about 30 seconds, then return it to the pan.

Options: If using the rosemary and/or garlic, add them immediately after all the liquid has been incorporated into the gravy. If you add the nutmeg and onion to the base recipe once the gravy starts simmering, you've got a classic French béchamel sauce.

Per ½-cup serving: 90 calories, 5 g protein, 12 g carbohydrate, 0.5 g sugar, 2 g total fat, 22% calories from fat, 2 g fiber, 315 mg sodium

—*JW*

Chimichurri Sauce

Makes about ¼ cup

This is a potent addition to any hearty dish and intensifies the flavor of any recipe it's added to. Use it sparingly, the way you might use mustard on a sandwich.

¾ cup roughly chopped fresh parsley

3 tablespoons white wine vinegar

2 tablespoons water

3 whole cloves garlic, peeled

⅛ teaspoon sea salt

½ teaspoon freshly ground black pepper

Optional: 2 tablespoons roasted diced green chiles or 1 diced fresh jalapeño; 1 tablespoon fresh oregano leaves; squeeze of fresh lime juice

Combine all the ingredients in a blender (including any optional ingredients) and blend until completely smooth.

Per ¼-cup serving: 29 calories, 1 g protein, 4 g carbohydrate, 0.3 g sugar, 0.2 g total fat, 25% calories from fat, 0.8 g fiber, 327 mg sodium

—JW

Spreads, Dips, and Snacks

Peach Salsa and Baked Pita Chips

Makes about 2 cups salsa (4 servings)

This flavorful salsa will be a hit at your next party!

1½ cups diced peaches
¼ cup diced red onion
¼ cup finely diced red bell pepper
2 tablespoons chopped fresh cilantro
1 tablespoon seeded minced jalapeño chile
Juice of 2 limes
⅛ teaspoon sea salt
4 whole-wheat pita breads, cut into 4 pieces and pulled apart

Preheat the oven to 350°F.

In a medium bowl, combine the peaches, onion, bell pepper, cilantro, jalapeño, lime juice, and salt. Cover and refrigerate for 1 hour before serving.

To make the pita chips, place the pita bread wedges on a baking sheet and bake for 5 minutes, or until crisp. Remove from the oven and cool, then serve with the salsa.

Per serving (¼ of recipe): 155 calories, 5 g protein, 33 g carbohydrate, 10 g sugar, 1 g total fat, 8% calories from fat, 5 g fiber, 314 mg sodium

—CW

White Bean Pâté

Makes about 2 cups (4 servings)

Serve this delicious dip with your favorite raw veggies for a healthy snack.

1 unpeeled onion, cut in half
1 15-ounce can low-sodium white beans, drained and rinsed
2 cloves garlic, minced
1½ tablespoons balsamic vinegar
Sea salt and freshly ground black pepper

Preheat the oven to 350°F.

Place the onion cut side down in a small baking dish. Bake for 1 hour, or until the onion is very soft and the skin slips off easily.

Place the cooked onion, beans, garlic, and vinegar in a blender or food processor. Blend, adding a little water as needed, until smooth. Season with salt and pepper to taste. Transfer to a bowl, cover, and refrigerate for 1 hour. Serve with celery sticks, carrot sticks, or whatever vegetables you enjoy.

Per serving (½ cup): 119 calories, 7 g protein, 22 g carbohydrate, 2 g sugar, 0.3 g total fat, 2% calories from fat, 5 g fiber, 371 mg sodium

—CW

Jicama Sticks with Orange Roasted Red Pepper Dip

Serves 1

Jicama (pronounced *HICK-uh-muh*) is a root veggie with a crisp, refreshing taste. Serve with the citrus roasted red pepper dip here or a simple sweet mustard.

½ small jicama, peeled

Juice of 1 orange

Juice of 1 lime

2 tablespoons fresh cilantro leaves

2 roasted red peppers

Pinch of sea salt

Cut the jicama in half (use half for this recipe and save the other half for more snacks or a salad later in the week). Slice the jicama ½ inch thick, then lay the slices flat and cut them into sticks.

Combine the orange juice, lime juice, cilantro, roasted red peppers, and salt in a food processor and process until smooth. Serve the dip with the jicama sticks.

Tip: When peeling the jicama, it's easier to use a paring knife than a vegetable peeler, as you'll want to slice about ¼ inch into the jicama in order to remove all the hard, rough skin.

Per serving: 170 calories, 4 g protein, 39 g carbohydrate, 21 g sugar, 0.9 g total fat, 5% calories from fat, 14 g fiber, 163 mg sodium

—JW

Mango and Watermelon with Lime

Serves 1

Fresh fruit dressed with lime juice and a touch of chili powder is a common snack throughout Mexico. The sourness of the lime juice coupled with the sweetness of the fruit gives the snack a nice pucker, and the chili powder adds zing!

1 mango, peeled, pitted, and sliced
2 wedges of watermelon
Juice of 1 lime
Sprinkling of chili powder

Slice the mango in half around the pit. Slice the mango into strips in the skin without piercing the skin. Scoop out the mango slices with a spoon. Sprinkle lime juice and chili powder on each slice of mango and wedge of watermelon.

Tip: Mangoes have a long, thin pit that runs down the length of the fruit. Slice just off the center of the mango, and if you hit the pit, gently run your knife along the side to get the most out of your mango. You may find it easier and safer to put the mango on a cutting board before you start slicing.

Per serving: 307 calories, 5 g protein, 79 g carbohydrate, 66 g sugar, 2 g total fat, 5% calories from fat, 6 g fiber, 110 mg sodium

—JW

Desserts

Banana Ice Cream

Makes 4 servings

If you're wondering where the other ingredients are in this recipe, there actually is only one—bananas! You have to try it to believe it!

8 ripe bananas

Peel and slice the bananas, place them in a container, cover, and freeze for at least 1 hour, until frozen. Remove the frozen bananas from the freezer and let them thaw a little at room temperature for 5 minutes. Place the bananas in a food processor and process until smooth and creamy, like soft-serve ice cream. You can vary the recipe by adding a little cinnamon, vanilla, or cocoa powder.

Per serving (¼ of recipe): 210 calories, 3 g protein, 54 g carbohydrate, 29 g sugar, 0.8 g total fat, 3% calories from fat, 6 g fiber, 2 mg sodium

—CW

Mom's Applesauce Cake

Serves 8

This moist spice cake has just the right level of sweetness and is perfect on an autumn afternoon. Thanks, Mom!

¼ teaspoon safflower oil
2 cups whole-wheat pastry flour, sifted
2 teaspoons aluminum-free baking powder
2 teaspoons baking soda
¼ teaspoon sea salt
2 teaspoons ground cinnamon
¼ teaspoon ground nutmeg
1⅓ cups unsweetened applesauce
1 cup rice milk
1 teaspoon pure vanilla extract
½ cup maple syrup
¾ cup raisins

Preheat the oven to 350°F and grease a 10-inch glass pie plate with the safflower oil.

In a large bowl, combine the flour, baking powder, baking soda, salt, cinnamon, and nutmeg and lightly stir with a whisk to aerate.

In a separate large bowl, combine the applesauce, rice milk, vanilla, and maple syrup and whisk to blend. Pour the wet ingredients into the dry ingredients and mix well. Add the raisins and stir to combine.

Pour the batter into the prepared pie plate and bake for 40 to 45 minutes, until the center springs back to the touch and a toothpick inserted in the center comes out clean. Cool in the pan completely before slicing and serving.

Per serving (⅛ of recipe): 243 calories, 5 g protein, 57 g carbohydrate, 27 g sugar, 1 g total fat, 4% calories from fat, 5 g fiber, 528 mg sodium

—CW

Fruity Couscous Cake

Serves 6

Great news—a cake you don't have to bake!

    4 cups apple juice
    1 teaspoon pure vanilla extract
    Pinch of sea salt
    2 cups uncooked couscous (the light-colored variety)
    2 cups blueberries
    ½ cup all-fruit jam
    1½ cups fresh fruit of your choice, for garnish (such as sliced
       peaches, kiwis, or strawberries)

In a medium saucepan, combine the apple juice, vanilla, and salt. Bring to a boil and add the couscous. Stir, cover, and reduce the heat to low; simmer for about 2 minutes. Turn off the heat and set aside, covered, for 5 to 10 minutes, until the juice has been absorbed. Gently fold the blueberries into the cooked couscous.

Rinse but don't dry a 9½-inch tart pan. Pour the couscous mixture into it and smooth the top with a spatula. Place the cake in the refrigerator and chill for at least 2 hours or until firm. Spread the jam over the cake and arrange the fresh fruit in a pretty pattern over the top.

Note: This cake can be made gluten free by replacing the couscous with uncooked polenta (corn grits). If using the polenta, increase the cooking time to 10 minutes.

Per serving (⅙ of recipe): 412 calories, 9 g protein, 93 g carbohydrate, 38 g sugar, 1 g total fat, 2% calories from fat, 7 g fiber, 72 mg sodium

—*CW*

Blackberry Bars

Makes 9 bars

These little jam squares are supereasy to make and filled with vitamin C–rich berries.

¼ teaspoon safflower oil
¾ cup barley flour, or flour of your choice
½ teaspoon sea salt
3 cups quick-cooking rolled oats
⅔ cup unsweetened applesauce
½ cup maple syrup
1 teaspoon pure vanilla extract
1 cup all-fruit blackberry jam

Preheat the oven to 350°F and lightly oil an 8 x 8-inch baking dish.

In a large bowl, combine the flour, salt, and oats.

In a small bowl, mix together the applesauce, maple syrup, and vanilla. Add the wet ingredients to the dry ingredients and mix well.

Cover the bottom of the prepared baking dish with half of the dough and press it until smooth. Spread the jam on top and crumble the remaining dough over the jam. Place in the oven and bake for 30 minutes, or until lightly golden on top. Cool in the pan and cut into bars.

Per serving (1 bar): 289 calories, 5 g protein, 64 g carbohydrate, 30 g sugar, 2 g total fat, 7% calories from fat, 7 g fiber, 139 mg sodium

—*CW*

Warm Apple Cherry Compote

Makes 4 servings

This simple dessert can be served in endless variations. Feel free to change up the fruits for fun, and top with a little low-fat granola for a delicious treat.

3 apples, cored and chopped
1 cup fresh or frozen and thawed pitted cherries
¼ cup apple juice
Pinch of sea salt
2 tablespoons maple syrup
1½ tablespoons cornstarch diluted in 2 tablespoons cold water
½ teaspoon ground cinnamon
1 teaspoon pure vanilla extract

Combine the apples, cherries, apple juice, salt, and maple syrup in a medium saucepan. Cover and bring to a gentle boil over medium-high heat. Reduce the heat to low and simmer, covered, for 5 minutes, or until the fruit is soft.

Slowly add the diluted cornstarch, stirring constantly to prevent lumping, until the mixture becomes thick. Stir in the cinnamon and vanilla and turn off the heat. Serve warm (or refrigerate and serve chilled).

Note: Kudzu root starch can be used in place of the cornstarch for an even healthier dessert. Kudzu is known for its alkalizing effects.

Per serving (¼ of recipe): 144 calories, 0.8 g protein, 37 g carbohydrate, 27 g sugar, 0.4 g total fat, 2% calories from fat, 4 g fiber, 77 mg sodium

—CW

Baked Fruit Compote

Makes 4 servings

This is a nice way to enjoy fruit. The spices and the baking transform simple fruit into a fat-free treat!

4 cups sliced peaches
1 cup blueberries

½ cup red raspberries
5 tablespoons maple syrup
½ teaspoon ground cinnamon
¼ teaspoon ground allspice
¼ teaspoon ground ginger
¼ teaspoon ground cloves

Preheat the oven to 350°F.

Combine all the ingredients in a large bowl and mix gently. Pour the fruit into a 2-quart baking dish, cover, and bake for 30 minutes, or until the fruit is soft. Serve warm.

Per serving (¼ of recipe): 150 calories, 2 g protein, 39 g carbohydrate, 32 g sugar, 0.7 g total fat, 4% calories from fat, 4 g fiber, 3 mg sodium

—CW

Minted Fruit Kebabs

Makes 4 kebabs (4 servings)

Fresh fruit makes a striking appearance in these antioxidant-rich kebabs. Enjoy them for a refreshing, light dessert!

8 red or green grapes
4 large strawberries
4 1-inch-square cantaloupe chunks
4 1-inch-square honeydew chunks
4 ½-inch-thick slices peeled kiwi
4 1-inch-square watermelon chunks
¼ cup orange juice
2 teaspoons fresh lime juice
2 tablespoons finely chopped fresh mint leaves
1 teaspoon pure vanilla extract
4 10-inch bamboo skewers

Thread 1 grape, 1 strawberry, 1 cantaloupe chunk, 1 honeydew chunk, 1 slice kiwi, 1 watermelon chunk, and 1 more grape onto a skewer. Repeat with the remaining fruit and skewers. Place the finished skewers in a shallow container.

In a small bowl, whisk together the orange juice, lime juice, mint, and vanilla. Pour the marinade over the fruit kebabs, cover, and chill

for at least 30 minutes (or up to 3 hours) in the refrigerator before
serving.

Per serving (1 kebab): 35 calories, 0.6 g protein, 8 g carbohydrate,
7 g sugar, 0.2 g total fat, 5% calories from fat, 1 g fiber, 5 mg sodium

—CW

Fruit Pops

Makes 6 pops

Now you can enjoy an all-natural frozen treat on those hot summer
days!

About 3 cups unsweetened fruit juice of your choice, such as
grape, pomegranate, or orange juice

Fill an ice pop mold (set of 6) with the juice and freeze for at least
3 hours. To remove a frozen pop from the mold, run briefly under
warm water.

Note: For variety, you can also use fruit juice concentrate such as
apple or orange blended with bananas, or add fresh berries or
chopped fresh fruit to the pops.

Per serving (1 pop): 76 calories, 0.5 g protein, 19 g carbohydrate,
18 g sugar, 0.2 g total fat, 2% calories from fat, 0.3 g fiber, 6 mg
sodium

—CW

Vanilla Berry Sorbet

Serves 4

This refreshing sorbet makes a light finish to any meal.

2 cups fresh or frozen raspberries or strawberries
¼ cup maple syrup or agave nectar, plus more if needed
1 teaspoon pure vanilla extract
Optional: ⅛ teaspoon almond extract

In a blender, combine all the ingredients and blend until smooth.
Adjust the sweetness to taste, if needed. Pour into a freezer
container, cover, and freeze for at least 3 hours, until firm. To serve,

remove the sorbet from freezer and let stand at room temperature until soft enough to scoop out.

Per serving (¼ of recipe): 88 calories, 0.7 g protein, 21 g carbohydrate, 15 g sugar, 0.4 g total fat, 4% calories from fat, 4 g fiber, 3 mg sodium

—CW

Super Raspberry Protein Brownies
Makes 16 brownies

A brownie made with beans? You bet! The beans add fiber, calcium, and protein, making these brownies a nutritious indulgence.

¼ teaspoon safflower oil
2 15-ounce cans low-sodium black beans, drained and rinsed
1 cup pitted dates
1 cup all-fruit raspberry jam
1 tablespoon pure vanilla extract
¼ cup whole-wheat pastry flour
1 cup unsweetened cocoa powder
¼ teaspoon sea salt

Preheat the oven to 350°F and grease an 9 x 9-inch baking pan with the oil.

Combine the black beans, dates, jam, and vanilla in a food processor and process until smooth. Add the flour, cocoa powder, and salt and process again to a stiff consistency, adding flour if necessary.

Pour into the prepared pan and smooth the top with a spatula. Bake for 30 minutes or until the top looks set. Remove from the oven and cool completely, then cut into 16 squares. The brownies will keep, refrigerated in a covered container, for up to 1 week.

Per serving (1 brownie): 145 calories, 5 g protein, 33 g carbohydrate, 15 g sugar, 1 g total fat, 7% calories from fat, 8 g fiber, 110 mg sodium

—CW

Baked Apples

Serves 4

Enjoy this warm and cozy dessert on a chilly night.

¼ teaspoon safflower oil
4 apples, peeled, cored, and sliced
¼ cup raisins
¼ cup rice milk
¼ cup maple syrup
2 tablespoons whole-wheat pastry flour
1 teaspoon ground cinnamon
¼ teaspoon ground nutmeg

Preheat the oven to 350°F and grease a 1½-quart casserole dish with the oil.

Combine the remaining ingredients in a large bowl and gently stir to coat the apple slices. Transfer to the prepared casserole dish and bake for 1 hour, or until the apples are soft. Serve warm.

Per serving (¼ of recipe): 182 calories, 1 g protein, 46 g carbohydrate, 34 g sugar, 0.9 g total fat, 4% calories from fat, 3 g fiber, 9 mg sodium

—CW

Chocolate Pudding

Serves 4

This creamy pudding is high in protein from the secret ingredient: beans!

1 15-ounce can low-sodium black beans, drained and rinsed
½ cup unsweetened cocoa powder
3 tablespoons maple syrup
3 tablespoons rice milk
1 teaspoon vanilla extract
¼ teaspoon sea salt
4 fresh raspberries, for garnish
4 mint sprigs, for garnish

Place all the ingredients in a blender or food processor and blend until smooth. Divide among individual serving glasses and chill for at least 1 hour before serving. Just before serving, garnish each glass with a raspberry and a mint sprig.

Per serving (¼ of recipe): 176 calories, 8 g protein, 37 g carbohydrate, 10 g sugar, 2 g total fat, 10% calories from fat, 11 g fiber, 294 mg sodium

—CW

Spiced Pumpkin Bread

Makes 1 loaf (12 slices)

This moist, satisfying bread will leave you wanting more. Go ahead… it's fat-free and sugar-free!

    2 cups whole-wheat pastry flour, sifted
    1 teaspoon aluminum-free baking powder
    1 teaspoon baking soda
    ¼ teaspoon sea salt
    1½ tablespoons flaxseed meal
    1 teaspoon ground cinnamon
    ⅛ teaspoon ground ginger
    ½ teaspoon pumpkin pie spice
    ½ cup rice milk
    1 cup plus 2 tablespoons canned pumpkin puree
    ½ cup maple syrup
    ½ teaspoon brown rice vinegar
    1 teaspoon pure vanilla extract
    ½ cup raisins

Preheat the oven to 350°F and grease a 1½-quart loaf pan.

In a large bowl, combine the flour, baking powder, baking soda, salt, flaxseed meal, cinnamon, ginger, and pumpkin pie spice and stir with a whisk to aerate.

In a medium bowl, whisk together the rice milk, pumpkin puree, maple syrup, vinegar, and vanilla. Add the wet ingredients to the dry ingredients and stir well. Fold in the raisins and pour the mixture evenly into the prepared loaf pan.

Bake for 1 hour, or until the center springs back to the touch and a toothpick inserted comes out clean. Cool thoroughly before slicing. Store in a covered container.

Per serving (1 slice): 140 calories, 3 g protein, 32 g carbohydrate, 13 g sugar, 1 g total fat, 6% calories from fat, 4 g fiber, 203 mg sodium

—CW

Lemon Rice

Serves 2

This recipe is similar to rice pudding but not nearly as sweet. The sweetness comes from the currants and almond milk, and the lemon juice adds a bit of brightness.

Juice of 1 lemon
¾ cup sweetened almond milk
½ teaspoon ground cinnamon
2 tablespoons currants
¼ cup short-grain brown rice
Zest of 1 lemon
Optional: 1 mango, peeled, pitted, and sliced

Zest a lemon and then juice it. Combine the almond milk, lemon juice, cinnamon, and currants in a medium saucepan and bring to a boil. Stir in the rice. Bring the liquid back to a boil, cover the pot, reduce the heat to low, and cook until the rice is soft, about 20 minutes. There should still be a bit of liquid left in the pot.

Divide the rice between serving bowls and top with the lemon zest.

Option: If you use the mango, add it before the lemon zest.

Tips: To zest a lemon, you'll need a zester or Microplane grater. Scrape the lemon deep enough that you take the peel of the lemon off the fruit but not so far that you dig into the whitish, bitter pith. The peel, not the pith, is the zest. To juice a lemon by hand, slice the lemon along a diagonal to expose as much surface area as possible while still being able to get a hand around the lemon. Squeeze the lemon with your hand, but have the cut side of the lemon facing toward your palm and let the juice run between your fingers, using your fingers as a makeshift sieve.

To slice a mango, see page 247.

Per serving (½ of recipe): 154 calories, 2 g protein, 32 g carbohydrate, 14 g sugar, 2 g total fat, 10% calories from fat, 1 g fiber, 62 mg sodium

—*JW*

Iced Watermelon and White Peach
Serves 8

This dish is the perfect refreshment for a hot day.

2 cups pureed white peaches
2 cups pureed watermelon
½ cup agave nectar
Optional: leaves from 1 small sprig of mint, preferably lemon mint

Remove the stems and pits from the peaches. Remove the seeds and rind from the watermelon. Place the peaches in the blender and puree them, then add the watermelon to the blender and puree again. Add the agave nectar and blend to incorporate.

Option: If you are using the mint, crush the mint with the back of a knife and puree it along with the peaches. Place the pureed mixture in a shallow metal or glass bowl and leave it in the freezer until it ices over. With a large metal spoon, scrape the frozen mixture to create a shaved ice treat.

Per serving (⅛ of recipe): 106 calories, 1 g protein, 27 g carbohydrate, 25 g sugar, 0.3 g total fat, 3% calories from fat, 1 g fiber, 1 mg sodium

—*JW*

Medications and Supplements to Treat Memory Problems

This book focuses on foods, exercise, and other steps that can prevent memory problems. But there are also medications and supplements that are used to try to reverse memory problems. For the most part, their effects are modest.

Here are the treatments that are commonly used or are now under active study.

Cholinesterase Inhibitors

A group of drugs called *cholinesterase inhibitors* boost the brain chemical *acetylcholine* and aim to slow the progression of Alzheimer's disease. Their effect is usually small. For about half of people whose condition is in the mild to moderate range, they delay worsening of symptoms by six months to one year. Approved cholinesterase inhibitors include:

donepezil (Aricept)
rivastigmine (Exelon)

galantamine (Razadyne)

tacrine (Cognex)

Tacrine was the first to be developed, but is rarely prescribed nowadays because of its ability to cause liver problems. Donepezil is approved by the Food and Drug Administration for all stages of Alzheimer's disease. Rivastigmine and galantamine are approved to treat mild to moderate cases.

These medications are generally safe but occasionally cause loss of appetite, nausea, vomiting, diarrhea, dizziness, confusion, and heart arrhythmia.

Memantine

Newer than the cholinesterase inhibitors, memantine (Namenda) works by blocking the action of a neurotransmitter called glutamate. It can be used in combination with cholinesterase inhibitors. However, so far memantine's benefits are not impressive. In 2011, researchers from the University of Southern California analyzed the results of three prior research studies, finding little evidence of benefit in mild to moderate Alzheimer's disease.[1] The drug can occasionally cause dizziness, confusion, headaches, and constipation.

Nasal Insulin

Insulin inhaled through the nose is being studied as a treatment for people with mild cognitive impairment or Alzheimer's disease. If this sounds surprising, there actually are good reasons to think it might help.

First, people with diabetes are at higher risk of developing Alzheimer's disease, and the key problem in diabetes is that insulin is malfunctioning or absent. It also turns out that insulin plays important roles in the brain. It helps build the synapses that link one cell to another and protects synapses from the effects of beta-amyloid.

The reason for giving insulin through the nose is that it can quickly travel to specific parts of the brain without affecting the rest of the body. So it does not affect your blood sugar the way an insulin injection would.

Researchers at the University of Washington in Seattle put it to the test. In a group of older volunteers with memory problems, the researchers did special brain scans to measure how well various parts of the brain were functioning. They also tested their memory by asking them to listen to a detailed story, then recall as much of it as they could twenty minutes later.[2] And they asked family members to rate how well the volunteers were doing.

They found that insulin treatment improved memory and protected the brain regions that were declining in untreated patients. The study was small and rather brief (four months); additional studies are under way to see how well insulin works over longer periods.

It is also worth remembering that the dietary approaches that are linked to reduced risk of Alzheimer's disease also help prevent and reverse diabetes.[3,4] As our research team showed several years ago, a low-fat, plant-based diet increases the body's sensitivity to insulin.[5]

Amyloid Immunotherapies

Researchers are testing methods to help the immune system clear away beta-amyloid from plaques in the brain. In this sort of treatment, an antibody is infused intravenously, triggering neighboring immune cells to engulf the amyloid and remove it.[6,7]

The good news is that these antibody treatments do indeed remove amyloid, which is an amazing achievement. The bad news is that removing amyloid has not so far been shown to significantly improve Alzheimer's symptoms. In other words, the patients' brain scans look better, but they remain impaired.

Researchers are hopeful that treatments of this type will eventually prove effective. In the meantime, the difficulty of developing these treatments reinforces the importance of a back-to-basics approach that looks at what habits predict Alzheimer's disease risk—high intake of saturated fat and metals, a lack of exercise, and so on—and focusing on changing those factors as early as possible.

Tau Phosphorylation and Aggregation Inhibitors

The neurofibrillary tangles that Alois Alzheimer first observed in brain cells in 1906 are now the targets of new medications.[8] They aim to prevent or reduce the changes in tau proteins that lead them to clump together.

These drugs have shown considerable promise in premarket testing, greatly slowing the decline in mental function in Alzheimer's patients without demonstrating severe side effects. However, studies with larger numbers of patients are needed to establish how effective and safe these treatments are.

Ginkgo Biloba

Ginkgo is an herbal extract commonly used as a memory booster. Derived from the leaves of the *Ginkgo biloba* tree, it is thought to be rich in antioxidants that protect the brain. The ginkgo tree itself is striking—it grows to a height of up to one hundred feet, and some trees are believed to be thousands of years old.

Unfortunately, ginkgo does not seem to prevent cognitive decline. Even though early studies did hold promise,[9] a team at the University of Pittsburgh and other research centers put ginkgo to a rigorous test. They brought in 3,069 people ages seventy-five and older and gave half of them ginkgo and the other half a placebo. The ginkgo dose was reasonably high—120 milligrams twice a day. But over the next six years, ginkgo proved a disappointment. It did nothing at all to prevent or delay the onset of memory problems or to slow the rate of cognitive decline.[10,11]

Could it help people who already have Alzheimer's? Most studies have shown no benefit.[12] This does not rule out the possibility that taking ginkgo over a longer period—perhaps starting early in life—might help. But based on these findings, it is hard to be optimistic about ginkgo.

If you do try ginkgo, it is important to know that it can interact with some commonly prescribed medications. It can add to the effect of blood thinners such as aspirin, ibuprofen, or warfarin, make antiseizure medications less effective, and accentuate the side effects of antidepressants. So even though it is an herbal preparation, it is essential to treat it like a drug and to speak with your physician before taking it.

Phosphatidylserine

Phosphatidylserine is a commonly sold nutritional supplement. Tests of its benefits for memory have yielded mixed results. Japanese researchers gave it to a group of elderly people with mild cognitive impairment to see if it would boost their memory.[13] It showed no benefit in people with mild memory problems, but did seem to help people with more serious memory deficits. A small study in Israel found much the same thing.[14] However, a larger study in the Netherlands found no benefits.[15] Bottom line—there's not yet much evidence favoring phosphatidylserine.

Chelation

Because metals—especially copper, iron, and zinc—have been found in the beta-amyloid plaques in the brains of people with Alzheimer's disease, researchers have looked for ways to remove these metals from the body. One method under study is chelation, which is already a standard treatment for heavy metal poisoning. Its name comes from the Greek word for "claw," referring to the ability of chelating chemicals to "grab" toxic molecules and remove them from the body.

A typical treatment involves administering a chelating agent, either orally or intravenously, and then allowing it to capture the offending toxin and carry it out through the kidneys into the urine. It is important to be very well hydrated, so as to avoid dangerous concentrations of the toxins as they pass through the kidneys.

Although chelation is well established for certain applications, such as lead or mercury poisoning, its use as an Alzheimer's treatment is still exploratory. Some findings have been promising, but we do not yet have enough information to know how helpful it might be.

So where does this leave us? Given the grave prognosis that Alzheimer's disease and other forms of dementia carry, it makes sense to push hard for effective treatments and to be rather liberal in putting treatments to use.

That said, the treatments that are currently available have been disappointing. If anything, they underscore the need for preventive steps so that treatments are not needed.

Ingredients That May Be New to You

Agave nectar (or agave syrup) Derived from the blue agave cactus, agave nectar is sweeter than table sugar, so you will find that you need less to achieve the same result. It is sold in many grocery stores and just about all health food stores.

Baking powder (aluminum-free) Typical brands of baking powder contain aluminum. Most stores stock one or more aluminum-free brands.

Buckwheat flour Despite its name, buckwheat is not actually related to wheat. But it is rich in complete protein and is used to make noodles, pancakes, and cereals. Because it is gluten-free, it is handy for people with celiac disease or gluten sensitivities.

Ener-G Egg Replacer This powdered mix of potato starch, tapioca starch, and leavening is sold at health food stores. Combined with water, it is a great binder, very much like eggs.

Flaxseed meal Flaxseed is rich in fiber and omega-3 fatty acids and has a slightly nutty taste. Flaxseed meal is often used as a binder in baked goods.

Hoisin sauce Found in the Asian aisle of grocery stores, hoisin sauce is a traditional Chinese dipping sauce.

Hummus A traditional Middle Eastern dish, this puree of chickpeas, tahini (sesame butter), garlic, and various flavorings serves as a breakfast food, sandwich filling, or dip. You will find it at most grocery stores.

Jicama Jicama is a large root that tastes a bit like an apple or pear. It can be added to salads or cut into sticks and served with dip.

Pepitas Pepitas are pumpkin seeds that usually are lightly roasted and used as a garnish.

Plantains Plantains are the fruit that make you do a double take in the produce aisle. They look like bananas but are a bit larger and firmer. Like bananas, they develop spots as they ripen.

Seitan Seitan (pronounced *SAY-tan*) is concentrated wheat protein, also called wheat gluten. It simulates a meaty texture in burgers and stir-fries. You will see it as an ingredient in commercial products and sold in shapes resembling meat at health food stores ready for you to add to dishes.

Soy sauce (low-sodium) Because most soy sauces are high in sodium, many companies provide brands that are modestly lower in sodium.

Tamari Many people prefer the rich flavor of tamari to other soy sauces. Unlike other varieties, tamari contains little or no wheat.

Tempeh Tempeh (pronounced *TEM-pay*) is made from soybeans that are fermented in a sturdy block. Sliced and marinated, it's a great substitute for hamburger, bacon, or sausage. It is found in health food stores.

Tofu Once known only to people in Asia, tofu is now available just about everywhere. Straight from the package, it is very much like cooked egg white. In your kitchen, it is extremely versatile, transforming into great substitutes for scrambled eggs, meat, cheese, and many other ingredients. You will find it in the produce aisle or in the refrigerator case, sold in water-packed boxes or convenient shelf-stable boxes.

Tomatillos As their name suggests, tomatillos are like little green tomatoes. They are used in Mexican sauces and salads.

Tomatoes, fire-roasted Roasted tomatoes add a special flavor to any dish you put them in. They are sold canned and are convenient to use.

Tomatoes, sun-dried Usually sold in the produce section, sun-dried tomatoes are a delicious addition to sauces, salads, and pizzas.

Whole-wheat pastry flour You might think it is only for pastries, but whole-wheat pastry flour has a fine texture that makes it perfect as a thickener and also as the basis for making flatbreads. It is available at health food stores and specialty markets.

References

Introduction

1. Epstein B. *A Cellarful of Noise.* Pocket Books, New York, 1967, 1998.

Chapter 1. Sharpen Your Memory, Enhance Your Brain

1. Albert MS, DeKosky ST, Dickson D, et al. The diagnosis of mild cognitive impairment due to Alzheimer's disease: Recommendations from the National Institute on Aging and Alzheimer's Association workgroup. *Alzheimers Dement.* 2011;7:270–79.

2. McKhann GM, Knopman DS, Chertkow H, et al. The diagnosis of dementia due to Alzheimer's disease: Recommendations from the National Institute on Aging and the Alzheimer's Association workgroup. *Alzheimers Dement.* 2011;7:263–69.

3. Farrer LA, Cupples LA, Haines JL, et al. Effects of age, sex, and ethnicity on the association between apolipoprotein E genotype and Alzheimer disease: A meta-analysis. APOE and Alzheimer Disease Meta Analysis Consortium. *JAMA.* 1997;278:1349–56.

4. Graff-Radford NR, Green RC, Go RC, et al. Association between apolipoprotein E genotype and Alzheimer disease in African American subjects. *Arch Neurol.* 2002;59:594–600.

5. Buchman AS, Leurgans SE, Nag S, Bennett DA, Schneider JA. Cerebrovascular disease pathology and parkinsonian signs in old age. *Stroke.* 2011;42:3183–89.

Chapter 2. Foods That Shield You from Toxic Metals

1. Lovell MA, Robertson JD, Teesdale WJ, Campbell JL, Markesbery WR. Copper, iron and zinc in Alzheimer's disease senile plaques. *J Neurol Sci.* 1998;158:47–52.

2. Stankiewicz JM, Brass SD. Role of iron in neurotoxicity: A cause for concern in the elderly? *Curr Opin Clin Nutr Metab Care.* 2009;12:22–29.

3. Salustri C, Barbati G, Ghidoni R, et al. Is cognitive function linked to serum free copper levels?: A cohort study in a normal population. *Clin Neurophysiol.* 2010;121:502–7.

4. Lam PK, Kritz-Silverstein D, Barrett-Connor E, et al. Plasma trace elements and cognitive function in older men and women: The Rancho Bernardo study. *J Nutrition.* 2008;12:22–27.

5. Morris MC, Evans DA, Tangney CC, et al. Dietary copper and high saturated and trans fat intakes associated with cognitive decline. *Arch Neurol.* 2006a;63:1085–88.

6. Brewer GJ. The risks of copper toxicity contributing to cognitive decline in the aging population and to Alzheimer's disease. *J Am Coll Nutr.* 2009;28:238–42.

7. Schiepers OJ, van Boxtel MP, de Groot RH, et al. Serum iron parameters, HFE C282Y genotype, and cognitive performance in older adults: Results from the FACIT study. *J Gerontol A Biol Sci Med Sci.* 2010;65:1312–21.

8. Shah RC, Wilson RS, Tang Y, Dong X, Murray A, Bennett DA. Relation of hemoglobin to level of cognitive function in older persons. *Neuroepidemiology.* 2009;32:40–46.

9. Shah RC, Buchman AS, Wilson RS, Leurgans SE, Bennett DA. Hemoglobin level in older persons and incident Alzheimer disease: Prospective cohort analysis. *Neurology.* 2011;77:219–26.

10. Huang X, Cuajungco MP, Atwood CS, Moir RD, Tanzi RE, Bush AI. Alzheimer's disease, beta-amyloid protein and zinc. *J Nutr.* 2000;130:1488S–92S.

11. Watt NT, Whitehouse IJ, Hooper NM. The role of zinc in Alzheimer's disease. *Int J Alzheimers Dis.* 2011;971021.

12. Smith MA, Harris PLR, Sayre LM, Perry G. Iron accumulation in Alzheimer's disease is a source of redox-generated free radicals. *Proc Nat Acad Sciences of the United States of America.* 1997;94:9866–68.

13. Environmental Protection Agency. Basic information about copper in drinking water. Internet: http://water.epa.gov/drink/contaminants/basicinformation/copper.cfm, accessed October 3, 2011.

14. Hunt JR. Bioavailability of iron, zinc, and other trace minerals from vegetarian diets. *Am J Clin Nutr.* 2003;78(suppl):633S–39S.

15. Hunt JR, Vanderpool RA. Apparent copper absorption from a vegetarian diet. *Am J Clin Nutr.* 2001;74:803–7.

16. Kadrabová J. Madaric A, Kováciková Z, Ginter E. Selenium status, plasma zinc, copper, and magnesium in vegetarians. *Biol Trace Elem Res.* 1995;50:13–24.

17. Crapper DR, Kishnan SS, Dalton AJ. Brain aluminum distribution in Alzheimer's disease and experimental neurofibrillary degeneration. *Science.* 1973;180:511–13.

18. Crapper DR, Krishnan SS, Quittkat S. Aluminium, neurofibrillary degeneration and Alzheimer's disease. *Brain.* 1976;99:67–80.

19. Miu AC, Benga O. Aluminum and Alzheimer's disease: A new look. *J Alzheimer's Dis.* 2006;10:179–201.

20. Bolognin S, Messori L, Drago D, Gabbiani C, Cendron L, Zatta P. Aluminum, copper, iron and zinc differentially alter amyloid-Aβ(1-42) aggregation and toxicity. *Int J Biochem Cell Biol.* 2011;43:877–85.

21. Martyn CN, Osmond C, Edwardson JA, Barker DJP, Harris EC, Lacey RF. Geographical relation between Alzheimer's disease and aluminium in drinking water. *Lancet.* 1989;333:61–62.

22. Rondeau V, Jacqmin-Gadda H, Commenges D, Helmer C, Dartigues J-F. Aluminum and silica in drinking water and the risk of Alzheimer's disease or cognitive decline: Findings from 15-year follow-up of the PAQUID cohort. *Am J Epidemiol.* 2009;169:489–96.

23. Frecker MF. Dementia in Newfoundland: Identification of a geographical isolate? *J Epidemiol Community Health.* 1991;45:307–11.

24. Gauthier E, Fortier I, Courchesne F, Pepin P, Mortimer J, Gauvreau D. Aluminum forms in drinking water and risk of Alzheimer's disease. *Environ Res.* 2000;84:234–46.

25. Forster DP, Newens AJ, Kay DW, Edwardson JA. Risk factors in clinically diagnosed presenile dementia of the Alzheimer type: A case-control study in northern England. *J Epidemiol Community Health.* 1995;49:253–58.

26. Taylor GA, Newens AJ, Edwardson JA, Kay DWK, Forster DP. Alzheimer's disease and the relationship between silicon and aluminum in water supplies in northern England. *J Epidemiol Community Health.* 1995;49: 323–28.

27. Forbes WF, McLachlan DR. Further thoughts on the aluminum-Alzheimer's disease link. *J Epidemiol Community Health.* 1996;50:401–3.

28. Doll R. Review: Alzheimer's disease and environmental aluminum. *Age Ageing.* 1993;22:138–53.

29. Alzheimer's Association. Alzheimer's Myths. Internet: http://www.alz.org/alzheimers_disease_myths_about_alzheimers.asp, accessed September 16, 2011.

30. Kawahara M, Kato-Negishi M. Link between aluminum and the pathogenesis of Alzheimer's disease: The integration of the aluminum and amyloid cascade hypotheses. *Int J Alzheimer's Dis.* 2011;276393.

31. Duggan JM, Dickeson JE, Tynan PF, Houghton A, Flynn JE. Aluminum beverage cans as a dietary source of aluminium. *Med J Aust.* 1992;156:604–5.

32. Saiyed SM, Yokel RA. Aluminium content of some foods and food products in the USA, with aluminium food additives. *Food Addit Contam.* 2005;22:234–44.

33. Mutter J, Naumann J, Schneider R, Walach H. Mercury and Alzheimer's disease. *Fortschr Neurol Psychiatr.* 2007;75:528–38.

34. Bates MN. Mercury amalgam dental fillings: An epidemiologic assessment. *Int J Hyg Environ Health.* 2006;209:309–16.

35. Saxe SR, Wekstein MW, Kryscio RJ, et al. Alzheimer's disease, dental amalgam and mercury. *J Am Dent Assoc.* 1999;130:191–99.

Chapter 3. Foods That Protect You from Harmful Fats and Cholesterol

1. Giem P, Beeson WL, Fraser GE. The incidence of dementia and intake of animal products: Preliminary findings from the Adventist Health Study. *Neuroepidemiology* 1993;12:28–36.

2. National Cancer Institute. Top food sources of saturated fat among US population, 2005–2006 NHANES. Internet: http://riskfactor.cancer.gov/diet/foodsources/sat_fat/sf.html, accessed October 2, 2011.

3. Morris MC, Evans EA, Bienias JL, et al. Dietary fats and the risk of incident Alzheimer's disease. *Arch Neurol.* 2003;60:194–200.

4. Luchsinger JA, Tang MX, Shea S, Mayeux R. Caloric intake and the risk of Alzheimer disease. *Arch Neurol.* 2002;59:1258–63.

5. Scarmeas N, Luchsinger JA, Schupf N, et al. Physical activity, diet, and risk of Alzheimer disease. *JAMA.* 2009;302:627–37.

6. Laitinen MH, Ngandu T, Rovio S, et al. Fat intake at midlife and risk of dementia and Alzheimer's disease: A population-based study. *Dement Geriatr Cogn Disord.* 2006;22:99–107.

7. Engelhart MJ, Geerlings MI, Ruitenberg A. Diet and risk of dementia: Does fat matter? The Rotterdam Study. *Neurology.* 2002;59:1915–21.

8. Solomon A, Kivipelto M, Wolozin B, Zhou J, Whitmer RA. Midlife serum cholesterol and increased risk of Alzheimer's and vascular dementia three decades later. *Dement Geriatr Cogn Disord.* 2009;28:75–80.

9. Puglielli L, Tanzi RE, Kovacs DM. Alzheimer's disease: The cholesterol connection. *Nature Neurosci.* 2003;6:345–51.

10. Anoop S, Anoop M, Meena K, Luthra K. Apolipoprotein E polymorphism in cerebrovascular & coronary heart diseases. *Indian J Med Res.* 2010;132:363–78.

11. Petot GJ, Traore F, Debanne SM, Lerner AJ, Smyth KA, Friedland RP. Interactions of apolipoprotein E genotype and dietary fat intake of healthy older persons during mid-adult life. *Metabolism.* 2003;52:279–81.

12. McGuinness B, Craig D, Bullock R, Passmore P. Statins for the prevention of dementia. *Cochrane Database Syst Rev.* 2009;15:CD003160.

13. Heude B, Ducimetiere P, Berre C, EVA Study. Cognitive decline and fatty acid composition of erythrocyte membranes—The EVA Study. *Am J Clin Nutr.* 2003;77:803–8.

14. Conquer JA, Tierney MC, Zecevic J, Bettger WJ, Fisher RH. Fatty acid analysis of blood plasma of patients with Alzheimer's disease, other types of dementia, and cognitive impairment. *Lipids.* 2000;35:1305–12.

15. Kröger E, Verreault R, Carmichael PH, et al. Omega-3 fatty acids and risk of dementia: The Canadian Study of Health and Aging. *Am J Clin Nutr.* 2009;90:184–92.

16. Davis BC, Kris-Etherton PM. Achieving optimal essential fatty acid status in vegetarians: Current knowledge and practical implications. *Am J Clin Nutr.* 2003;78(suppl):640S–46S.

17. Dangour AD, Allen E, Elbourne D, et al. Effect of 2-y n-3 long-chain polyunsaturated fatty acid supplementation on cognitive function in older people: A randomized, double-blind, controlled trial. *Am J Clin Nutr.* 2010;91:1725–32.

18. Van de Rest O, Geleijnse JM, Kok FJ, et al. Effect of fish oil on cognitive performance in older subjects: A randomized, controlled trial. *Neurology.* 2008;71:430–38.

19. Quinn JF, Rama R, Thomas RG, et al. Docosahexaenoic acid supplementation and cognitive decline in Alzheimer disease: A randomized trial. *JAMA.* 2010;304:1903–11.

20. Morris MC, Evans DA, Tangney CC, Bienias JL, Wilson RS. Fish consumption and cognitive decline with age in a large community study. *Arch Neurol.* 2005;62:1849–53.

21. Tangney CC, Kwasny MJ, Li H, Wilson RS, Evans DA, Morris MC. Adherence to a Mediterranean-type dietary pattern and cognitive decline in a community population. *Am J Clin Nutr.* 2011;93:601–7.

22. Tonstad S, Butler T, Yan R, Fraser GE. Type of vegetarian diet, body weight and prevalence of type 2 diabetes. *Diabetes Care.* 2009;32:791–96.

23. Marckmann P, Grønbaek M. Fish consumption and coronary heart disease mortality: A systematic review of prospective cohort studies. *Eur J Clin Nutr.* 1999;53:585–90.

24. Féart C, Samieri C, Rondeau V, et al. Adherence to a Mediterranean diet, cognitive decline, and risk of dementia. *JAMA.* 2009;302:638–48.

25. Barnard ND, Scialli AR, Turner-McGrievy G, Lanou AJ, Glass J. The effects of a low-fat, plant-based dietary intervention on body weight, metabolism, and insulin sensitivity. *Am J Med.* 2005;118:991–97.

26. Berkow S, Barnard ND. Vegetarian diets and weight status. *Nutr Rev.* 2006;64:175–88.

27. Turner-McGrievy GM, Barnard ND, Scialli AR. A two-year randomized weight loss trial comparing a vegan diet to a more moderate low-fat diet. *Obesity.* 2007;15:2276–81.

28. Gustafson D. An 18-year follow-up of overweight and risk of Alzheimer's disease. *Arch Intern Med.* 2003;163:1524–28.

29. Berkow S, Barnard ND. Blood pressure regulation and vegetarian diets. *Nutr Rev.* 2005;63:1–8.

Chapter 4. Foods That Build Your Vitamin Shield

1. Devore EE, Grodstein F, van Rooij FJ, Hofman A, Stampfer MJ, Witteman JC, Breteler MM. Dietary antioxidants and long-term risk of dementia. *Arch Neurol.* 2010;67:819–25.

2. Morris MC, Evans DA, Bienias JL, Tangney CC, Bennett DA, Aggarwal N, Wilson RS, Scherr PA. Dietary intake of antioxidant nutrients and the risk of incident Alzheimer disease in a biracial community study. *JAMA.* 2002;287:3230–37.

3. Morris MC, Evans DA, Tangney CC, et al. Relation of the tocopherol forms to incident Alzheimer disease and cognitive change. *Am J Clin Nutr.* 2005;81:508–14.

4. Laurin D, Foley DJ, Masaki KH, White LR, Launer LJ. Vitamin E and C supplements and risk of dementia. *JAMA.* 2002;288:2266–68.

5. Sano M, Ernesto C, Thomas RG, et al. A controlled trial of selegiline, alpha-tocopherol, or both as treatment for Alzheimer's disease. The Alzheimer's Disease Cooperative Study. *N Engl J Med.* 1997;336:1216–22.

6. Thomas RG, Gebhardt SE. Nuts and seeds as sources of alpha and gamma tocopherols. USDA-ARS Nutrient Data Laboratory, Beltsville, MD. Internet: http://www.ars.usda.gov/SP2UserFiles/Place/12354500/Articles/AICR06 _NutSeed.pdf, accessed June 17, 2011.

7. Brewer GJ. The risks of copper toxicity contributing to cognitive decline in the aging population and to Alzheimer's disease. *J Am Coll Nutr.* 2009;28:238–42.

8. Durga J, van Boxtel MP, Schouten EG, et al. Effect of 3-year folic acid supplementation on cognitive function in older adults in the FACIT trial: A randomised, double blind, controlled trial. *Lancet.* 2007a;369:208–16.

9. de Jager CA, Oulhaj A, Jacoby R, Refsum H, Smith AD. Cognitive and clinical outcomes of homocysteine-lowering B-vitamin treatment in mild cognitive impairment: A randomized controlled trial. *Int J Geriatr Psychiatry.* 2011; Jul 21. doi: 10.1002/gps.2758. [Epub ahead of print]

10. Durga J, Verhoef P, Anteunis LJ, Schouten E, Kok FJ. Effects of folic acid supplementation on hearing in older adults: A randomized, controlled trial. *Ann Intern Med.* 2007b;146:1–9.

11. Ravaglia G, Forti P, Maioli F, Martelli M, Servadei L, Brunetti N, Porcellini E, Licastro F. Homocysteine and folate as risk factors for dementia and Alzheimer disease. *Am J Clin Nutr.* 2005;82:636–43.

12. Tucker KL, Qiao N, Scott T, Rosenberg I, Spiro A 3rd. High homocysteine and low B vitamins predict cognitive decline in aging men: The Veterans Affairs Normative Aging Study. *Am J Clin Nutr.* 2005;82:627–35.

13. Aisen PS, Schneider LS, Sano M, et al. High-dose B vitamin supplementation and cognitive decline in Alzheimer's disease: A randomized controlled trial. *JAMA.* 2008;300:1774–83.

14. Ligthart SA, Moll van Charante EP, Van Gool WA, Richard E. Treatment of cardiovascular risk factors to prevent cognitive decline and dementia: A systematic review. *Vasc Health Risk Manag.* 2010;6:775–85.

15. Morris MC, Evans DA, Schneider JA, Tangney CC, Bienias JL, Aggarwal NT. Dietary folate and vitamins B-12 and B-6 not associated with incident Alzheimer's disease. *J Alzheimer's Dis.* 2006a;9:435–43.

16. Bønaa KH, Njølstad I, Ueland PM, et al. Homocysteine lowering and cardiovascular events after acute myocardial infarction. *N Engl J Med.* 2006;354:1578–88.

17. Feng L, Li J, Yap KB, Kua EH, Ng TP. Vitamin B-12, apolipoprotein E genotype, and cognitive performance in community-living older adults: Evidence of a gene-micronutrient interaction. *Am J Clin Nutr.* 2009;89: 1263–68.

18. Morris MC, Evans DA, Tangney CC, Bienias JL, Wilson RS. Associations of vegetable and fruit consumption with age-related cognitive change. *Neurology.* 2006b;67:1370–76.

19. Dauchet L, Amouyel P, Dallongeville J. Fruit and vegetable consumption and risk of stroke: A meta-analysis of cohort studies. *Neurology.* 2005;65:1193–97.

20. He FJ, Nowson CA, MacGregor GA. Fruit and vegetable consumption and stroke: Meta-analysis of cohort studies. *Lancet.* 2006;367:320–26.

21. Oude Griep LM, Monique Verschuren WM, Kromhout D, Ocké MC, Geleijnse JM. Colours of fruit and vegetables and 10-year incidence of CHD. *Br J Nutr.* 2011a;106:1562–69.

22. Oude Griep LM, Vershuren WMM, Kromhout D, Ocke MC, Geleijnse JM. Colors of fruit and vegetables and 10-year incidence of stroke. *Stroke.* 2011b;42:3190–95.

23. Krikorian R, Nash TA, Shidler MD, Shukitt-Hale B, Joseph JA. Concord grape juice supplementation improves memory function in older adults with mild cognitive impairment. *Br J Nutr.* 2010;103:730–34.

24. Krikorian R, Shidler MD, Nash TA, et al. Blueberry supplementation improves memory in older adults. *J Agric Food Chem.* 2010;58:3996–4000.

25. Letenneur L. Risk of dementia and alcohol and wine consumption: A review of recent results. *Biol Res.* 2004;37:189–93.

26. Ioannou GN, Dominitz JA, Weiss NS, Heagerty PJ, Kowdley KV. The effect of alcohol consumption on the prevalence of iron overload, iron deficiency, and iron deficiency anemia. *Gastroenterology.* 2004;126:1293–1301.

27. Eskelinen MH, Kivipelto M. Caffeine as a protective factor in dementia and Alzheimer's disease. *J Alzheimer's Dis.* 2010;20:S167–74.

Chapter 5. Mental Exercises That Build Your Cognitive Reserve

1. Rentz DM, Locascio JJ, Becker JA, et al. Cognition, reserve, and amyloid deposition in normal aging. *Ann Neurol.* 2010;67:353–64.

2. Yaffee K, Weston A, Graff-Radford NR. Association of plasma β-amyloid level and cognitive reserve with subsequent cognitive decline. *JAMA.* 2011; 305:261–66.

3. Wilson RS, Bennett DA, Bienias JL, et al. Cognitive activity and incident AD in a population-based sample of older persons. *Neurology.* 2002; 59:1910–14.

4. Willis SL, Tennstedt SL, Marsiske M, et al. Long-term effects of cognitive training on everyday functional outcomes in older adults. *JAMA.* 2006; 296:2805–14.

5. Jean L, Bergeron ME, Thivierge S, Simard M. Cognitive intervention programs for individuals with mild cognitive impairment: Systematic review of the literature. *Am J Geriatr Psychiatry.* 2010;18:281–96.

6. Craik FIM, Bialystok E, Freedman M. Delaying the onset of Alzheimer disease: Bilingualism as a form of cognitive reserve. *Neurology.* 2010; 75:1726–29.

7. Chertkow H, Whitehead V, Phillips N, Wolfwon C, Atherton J, Bergman H. Multilingualism (but not always bilingualism) delays the onset of Alzheimer disease: Evidence from a bilingual community. *Alzheimer Dis Assoc Discord.* 2010;24:118–25.

8. Kavé G, Eyal N, Shorek A, Cohen-Mansfield J. Multilingualism and cognitive state in the oldest old. *Psychol Aging.* 2008;23;70–78.

9. Inoue S, Matsuzawa T. Working memory of numerals in chimpanzees. *Curr Biol.* 2007;17(23):R1004–5.

10. Inoue S, Matsuzawa T. Acquisition and memory of sequence order in young and adult chimpanzees (Pan troglodytes). *Anim Cogn.* 2009;12,Suppl 1:S59–69.

Chapter 6. Physical Exercises That Protect Your Brain

1. Pereira AC, Huddleston DE, Brickman AM, et al. An in vivo correlate of exercise-induced neurogenesis in the adult dentate gyrus. *Proc Natl Acad Sci USA.* 2007;104:5638–43.

2. Colcombe SJ, Erickson KI, Scalf PE, et al. Aerobic exercise training increases brain volume in aging humans. *J. Gerontol A Biol Sci Med Sci.* 2006;61:1166–70.

3. Erickson KI, Voss MW, Prakash RS, et al. Exercise training increases size of hippocampus and improves memory. *Proc Natl Acad Sci USA.* 2011;108:3017–22.

4. Larson EB, Wang L, Bowen JD, et al. Exercise is associated with reduced risk for incident dementia among persons 65 years of age and older. *Ann Intern Med.* 2006;17:144:73–81.

5. Scarmeas N, Luchsinger JA, Schupf N, et al. Physical activity, diet, and risk of Alzheimer disease. *JAMA.* 2009;302:627–37.

6. Rovio S, Kareholt I, Helkala EL, et al. Leisure-time physical activity at midlife and the risk of dementia and Alzheimer's disease. *Lancet Neurology.* 2005;4:705–11.

7. Hamer M, Chida Y. Physical activity and risk of neurodegenerative disease: A systematic review of prospective evidence. *Psychol Med.* 2009;39:3–11.

8. Foster PP, Rosenblatt KP, Kuljis RO. Exercise-induced cognitive plasticity, implications for mild cognitive impairment and Alzheimer's disease. *Frontiers in Neurology.* 2011;2:1–15.

9. Voss MW, Chaddock L, Kim JS, et al. Aerobic fitness is associated with greater efficiency of the network underlying cognitive control in preadolescent children. *Neuroscience.* 2011;29;199:166–76.

10. Boulé NG, Haddad E, Kenny GP, Wells GA, Sigal RJ. Effects of exercise on glycemic control and body mass in type 2 diabetes mellitus: A meta-analysis of controlled clinical trials. *JAMA.* 2001;286:1218–27.

11. Curioni CC, Lourenco PM. Long-term weight loss after diet and exercise: A systematic review. *Int J Obes* (Lond) 2005;29:1168–74.

12. Colcombe SJ, Kramer AF, Erickson KI, et al. Cardiovascular fitness, cortical plasticity, and aging. *Proc Natl Acad Sci USA.* 2004;101:3316–21.

Chapter 7. Build Memory Power as You Sleep

1. Wagner U, Born J. Memory consolidation during sleep: Interactive effects of sleep stages and HPA regulation. *Stress*. 2008;11:28–41.
2. Huang Y, Potter R, Sigurdson W, et al. Effects of age and amyloid deposition on aß dynamics in the human central nervous system. *Arch Neurol*. 2012;69:51–58.

Chapter 8. Medicines and Health Conditions That Affect Memory

1. Preiss D, Seshasai SR, Welsh P, et al. Risk of incident diabetes with intensive-dose compared with moderate-dose statin therapy: A meta-analysis. *JAMA*. 2011;305:2556–64.
2. Evans MA, Golomb BA. Statin-associated adverse cognitive effects: Survey results from 171 patients. *Pharmacotherapy*. 2009;29:800–811.
3. Cherrier M, Amory J, Ersek M, Risler L, Shen D. Comparative cognitive and subjective side effects of immediate release oxycodone in healthy middle age and older adults. *J Pain*. 2009;10:1038–50.
4. Ockene JK, Barad DH, Cochrane BB, et al. Symptom experience after discontinuing use of estrogen plus progestin. *JAMA*. 2005;294:183–93.
5. Le Pira F, Zappalà G, Giuffrida S, et al. Memory disturbances in migraine with and without aura: A strategy problem? *Cephalalgia*. 2000;20:475–78.
6. Farmer K, Cady R, Bleiberg J, et al. Sumatriptan nasal spray and cognitive function during migraine: Results of an open-label study. *Headache*. 2001;41:377–84.
7. Brezden CB, Phillips KA, Abdolell M, Bunston T, Tannock IF. Cognitive function in breast cancer patients receiving adjuvant chemotherapy. *J Clin Oncol*. 2000;18:2695–701.
8. Dietrich J, Han R, Yang Y, Mayer-Pröschel M, Noble M. CNS progenitor cells and oligodendrocytes are targets of chemotherapeutic agents in vitro and in vivo. *J Biol*. 2006;5:22.
9. Ohara T, Doi Y, Ninomiya T, et al. Glucose tolerance status and risk of dementia in the community: The Hisayama study. *Neurology*. 2011;77:1126–34.

Chapter 9. A Brain-Enhancing Menu

1. Ornish D, Brown SE, Scherwitz LW, et al. Can lifestyle changes reverse coronary heart disease?: The Lifestyle Heart Trial. *Lancet*. 1990;336:129–33.

2. Ornish D, Scherwitz LW, Billings JH, et al. Intensive lifestyle changes for reversal of coronary heart disease. *JAMA*. 1998;280:2001–7.

3. Barnard ND, Scialli AR, Turner-McGrievy G, Lanou AJ, Glass J. The effects of a low-fat, plant-based dietary intervention on body weight, metabolism, and insulin sensitivity. *Am J Med*. 2005;118:991–97.

4. Barnard ND, Cohen J, Jenkins DJ, et al. A low-fat, vegan diet improves glycemic control and cardiovascular risk factors in a randomized clinical trial in individuals with type 2 diabetes. *Diabetes Care*. 2006;29:1777–83.

5. Tonstad S, Butler T, Yan R, Fraser GE. Type of vegetarian diet, body weight and prevalence of type 2 diabetes. *Diabetes Care*. 2009;32:791–96.

6. Anderson JW, Gustafson NJ, Spencer DB, Tietyen J, Bryant CA. Serum lipid response of hypercholesterolemic men to single and divided doses of canned beans. *Am J Clin Nutr*. 1990;51:1013–19.

7. Messina M, Messina V. *The Simple Soybean and Your Health*. Avery Publishing Group, Garden City Park, New York, 1994.

8. Mukuddem-Petersen J, Oosthuizen W, Jerling JC. A systematic review of the effects of nuts on blood lipid profiles in humans. *J Nutr*. 2005;135: 2082–89.

9. Jenkins DJ, Kendall CW, Marchie A, et al. Direct comparison of a dietary portfolio of cholesterol-lowering foods with a statin in hypercholesterolemic participants. *Am J Clin Nutr*. 2005;81:380–87.

10. Davis BC, Kris-Etherton P. Achieving optimal essential fatty acid status in vegetarians: Current knowledge and practical implications. *Am J Clin Nutr*. 2003;78(suppl):640S–46S.

Chapter 10. Conquer Food Cravings

1. David Sheff. Interview with John Lennon and Yoko Ono. *Playboy*, January 1981. Internet: http://www.beatlesinterviews.org/db1980.jlpb.beatles .html, accessed September 3, 2011.

2. Ray Coleman. *The Man Who Made the Beatles: An Intimate Biography of Brian Epstein*. McGraw Hill, New York, 1989, pp. 10–15, 318–41.

3. Yeomans MR, Wright P, Macleod HA, Critchley JAJH. Effects of nalmefene on feeding in humans. *Psychopharmacology*. 1990;100:426–32.

4. Barnard ND, Noble EP, Ritchie T, et al. D2 Dopamine receptor Taq1A polymorphism, body weight, and dietary intake in type 2 diabetes. *Nutrition*. 2009;25:58–65.

5. The Vegetarian. February 1992. Internet: http://www.eatveg.com/paul .htm, accessed November 6, 2011.

Appendix 1. Medications and Supplements to Treat Memory Problems

1. Schneider LS, Dagerman KS, Higgins JP, McShane R. Lack of evidence for the efficacy of memantine in mild Alzheimer disease. *Arch Neurol.* 2011; 68:991–98.

2. Craft S, Baker LD, Montine TJ, et al. Intranasal insulin therapy for Alzheimer disease and amnestic mild cognitive impairment. *Arch Neurol.* 2012;69:29–38.

3. Barnard ND, Cohen J, Jenkins DJ, et al. A low-fat, vegan diet improves glycemic control and cardiovascular risk factors in a randomized clinical trial in individuals with type 2 diabetes. *Diabetes Care.* 2006;29:1777–83.

4. Barnard ND, Cohen J, Jenkins DJ, et al. A low-fat vegan diet and a conventional diabetes diet in the treatment of type 2 diabetes: A randomized, controlled, 74-week clinical trial. *Am J Clin Nutr.* 2009;89(suppl):1588S–96S.

5. Barnard ND, Scialli AR, Turner-McGrievy G, Lanou AJ, Glass J. The effects of a low-fat, plant-based dietary intervention on body weight, metabolism, and insulin sensitivity. *Am J Med.* 2005;118:991–97.

6. Nicoll JAR, Wilkinson D, Holmes C, Steart P, Markham H, Weller RO. Neuropathology of human Alzheimer disease after immunization with amyloid-β peptide: A case report. *Nat Med.* 2003;9:448–52.

7. Ostrowitzki S, Deptula D, Thurfjell L, et al. Mechanism of amyloid removal in patients with Alzheimer disease treated with gantenerumab. *Arch Neurol.* Published online, October 10, 2011.

8. Badiola N, Suárez-Calvet M, Lleó A. Tau phosphorylation and aggregation as a therapeutic target in tauopathies. *CNS & Neurological Disorders—Drug Targets.* 2010;9:727–40.

9. Kanowski S, Hoerr R. Ginkgo biloba extract EGb 761 in dementia: Intent-to-treat analyses of a 24-week, multi-center, double-blind, placebo-controlled, randomized trial. *Pharmacopsychiatry.* 2003;36:297–303.

10. DeKosky ST, Williamson JD, Fitzpatrick AL, et al. Ginkgo biloba for prevention of dementia: A randomized controlled trial. *JAMA.* 2008; 300:2253–62.

11. Snitz BE, O'Meara ES, Carlson MC, et al. Ginkgo biloba for preventing cognitive decline in older adults: A randomized trial. *JAMA.* 2009;302: 2663–70.

12. Birks J, Grimley Evans J. Ginkgo biloba for cognitive impairment and dementia. *Cochrane Database Syst Rev.* 2009;21:CD003120.

13. Kato-Kataoka A, Sakai M, Ebina R, Nonaka C, Asano T, Miyamori T. Soybean-derived phosphatidylserine improves memory function of the

elderly Japanese subjects with memory complaints. *J Clin Biochem Nutr.* 2010;47:246–55.

14. Richter Y, Herzog Y, Cohen T, Steinhart Y. The effect of phosphatidylserine-containing omega-3 fatty acids on memory abilities in subjects with subjective memory complaints: A pilot study. *Clin Interv Aging.* 2010;5:313–16.

15. Jorissen BL, Brouns F, Van Boxtel MP, et al. The influence of soy-derived phosphatidylserine on cognition in age-associated memory impairment. *Nutritional Neuroscience.* 2001;4:121–34.

Index

About the Author

Neal D. Barnard, MD, leads research studies to improve the health of people with diabetes, obesity, and other serious health problems, and spearheads efforts to improve nutrition in schools and in the workplace. He is an adjunct associate professor of medicine at George Washington University in Washington, DC, and a Diplomat of the American Board of Psychiatry and Neurology. His groundbreaking research funded by the National Institutes of Health showed that nutrition can be more powerful than oral medicines for treating diabetes. Dr. Barnard received his MD degree at the George Washington University School of Medicine in Washington, DC, and completed his residency at the same institution. He practiced at St. Vincent's Hospital in New York before returning to Washington to found the Physicians Committee for Responsible Medicine (PCRM) in order to promote preventive medicine, to conduct clinical research, and to promote higher ethical standards in research.

Dr. Barnard's research studies have been cited by the American Diabetes Association and the American Dietetic Association in official policy statements on healthful diets. His articles have appeared in *Diabetes Care the American Journal of Clinical Nutrition,* the *American Journal of Medicine, Pediatrics,* the

Journal of the American Dietetic Association, Scientific American, the *American Journal of Cardiology, Obstetrics & Gynecology, Lancet Oncology, Preventive Medicine,* and many other scientific and medical journals. He is a frequent lecturer at scientific societies and a peer reviewer for many medical journals. He is a frequent guest on network television and has hosted three PBS programs—*Tackling Diabetes, Kickstart Your Health,* and *Protect Your Memory.* He is the author of the national bestsellers, *Dr. Neal Barnard's Program for Reversing Diabetes* and *21-Day Weight Loss Kickstart,* as well as fifteen other books.

Christine Waltermyer is the founder and director of The Natural Kitchen Cooking School, offering Chef Training Programs, personal chef service, and in-home cooking classes in Princeton, NJ, and Manhattan. With more than a decade of experience in the field of natural cooking, Christine is a masterful chef and teacher specializing in macrobiotic and vegan cuisines.

Jason Wyrick is the executive chef and publisher of the magazine, *The Vegan Culinary Experience.* Jason's work has been featured in the *New York Times,* and he has catered for companies such as Google, Frank Lloyd Wright Foundation, and Farm Sanctuary, and has been a guest instructor in the Le Cordon Bleu program at Scottsdale Culinary Institute. Jason supplied the recipes for Dr. Barnard's book, the *21-Day Weight Loss Kickstart.*